Minimally Invasive Urological Procedures and Related Technological Developments

Minimally Invasive Urological Procedures and Related Technological Developments

Editor

Bhaskar Somani

MDPI • Basel • Beijing • Wuhan • Barcelona • Belgrade • Manchester • Tokyo • Cluj • Tianjin

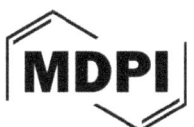

Editor
Bhaskar Somani
University of Southampton
UK

Editorial Office
MDPI
St. Alban-Anlage 66
4052 Basel, Switzerland

This is a reprint of articles from the Special Issue published online in the open access journal *Journal of Clinical Medicine* (ISSN 2077-0383) (available at: https://www.mdpi.com/journal/jcm/special_issues/Minimally_Invasive_Urological_Procedures).

For citation purposes, cite each article independently as indicated on the article page online and as indicated below:

LastName, A.A.; LastName, B.B.; LastName, C.C. Article Title. *Journal Name* **Year**, *Volume Number*, Page Range.

ISBN 978-3-0365-2708-6 (Hbk)
ISBN 978-3-0365-2709-3 (PDF)

Cover image courtesy of Bhaskar Somani

© 2021 by the authors. Articles in this book are Open Access and distributed under the Creative Commons Attribution (CC BY) license, which allows users to download, copy and build upon published articles, as long as the author and publisher are properly credited, which ensures maximum dissemination and a wider impact of our publications.

The book as a whole is distributed by MDPI under the terms and conditions of the Creative Commons license CC BY-NC-ND.

Contents

About the Editor vii

Bhaskar Somani
Special Issue 'Minimally Invasive Urological Procedures and Related Technological Developments'
Reprinted from: *J. Clin. Med.* **2021**, *10*, 4225, doi:10.3390/jcm10184225 1

Amelia Pietropaolo, Robert M. Geraghty, Rajan Veeratterapillay, Alistair Rogers, Panagiotis Kallidonis, Luca Villa, Luca Boeri, Emanuele Montanari, Gokhan Atis, Esteban Emiliani, Tarik Emre Sener, Feras Al Jaafari, John Fitzpatrick, Matthew Shaw, Chris Harding and Bhaskar K. Somani
A Machine Learning Predictive Model for Post-Ureteroscopy Urosepsis Needing Intensive Care Unit Admission: A Case–Control YAU Endourology Study from Nine European Centres
Reprinted from: *J. Clin. Med.* **2021**, *10*, 3888, doi:10.3390/jcm10173888 5

Wen-Ling Wu, Oluwaseun Adebayo Bamodu, Yuan-Hung Wang, Su-Wei Hu, Kai-Yi Tzou, Chi-Tai Yeh and Chia-Chang Wu
Extracorporeal Shockwave Therapy (ESWT) Alleviates Pain, Enhances Erectile Function and Improves Quality of Life in Patients with Chronic Prostatitis/Chronic Pelvic Pain Syndrome
Reprinted from: *J. Clin. Med.* **2021**, *10*, 3602, doi:10.3390/jcm10163602 15

Audrey Uzan, Paul Chiron, Frédéric Panthier, Mattieu Haddad, Laurent Berthe, Olivier Traxer and Steeve Doizi
Comparison of Holmium:YAG and Thulium Fiber Lasers on the Risk of Laser Fiber Fracture
Reprinted from: *J. Clin. Med.* **2021**, *10*, 2960, doi:10.3390/jcm10132960 29

Simone J. M. Stoots, Guido M. Kamphuis, Rob Geraghty, Liffert Vogt, Michaël M. E. L. Henderickx, B. M. Zeeshan Hameed, Sufyan Ibrahim, Amelia Pietropaolo, Enakshee Jamnadass, Sahar M. Aljumaiah, Saeed B. Hamri, Eugenio Ventimiglia, Olivier Traxer, Vineet Gauhar, Etienne X. Keller, Vincent De Coninck, Otas Durutovic, Nariman K. Gadzhiev, Laurian B. Dragos, Tarik Emre Sener, Nick Rukin, Michele Talso, Panagiotis Kallidonis, Esteban Emiliani, Ewa Bres-Niewada, Kymora B. Scotland, Naeem Bhojani, Athanasios Vagionis, Angela Piccirilli and Bhaskar K. Somani
Global Variations in the Mineral Content of Bottled Still and Sparkling Water and a Description of the Possible Impact on Nephrological and Urological Diseases
Reprinted from: *J. Clin. Med.* **2021**, *10*, 2807, doi:10.3390/jcm10132807 37

Amelia Pietropaolo, Thomas Hughes, Mriganka Mani and Bhaskar Somani
Outcomes of Ureteroscopy and Laser Stone Fragmentation (URSL) for Kidney Stone Disease (KSD): Comparative Cohort Study Using MOSES Technology 60 W Laser System versus Regular Holmium 20 W Laser
Reprinted from: *J. Clin. Med.* **2021**, *10*, 2742, doi:10.3390/jcm10132742 51

Sunil Pillai, Akshay Kriplani, Arun Chawla, Bhaskar Somani, Akhilesh Pandey, Ravindra Prabhu, Anupam Choudhury, Shruti Pandit, Ravi Taori and Padmaraj Hegde
Acute Kidney Injury Post-Percutaneous Nephrolithotomy (PNL): Prospective Outcomes from a University Teaching Hospital
Reprinted from: *J. Clin. Med.* **2021**, *10*, 1373, doi:10.3390/jcm10071373 57

Robert M. Geraghty, Paul Cook, Paul Roderick and Bhaskar Somani
Risk of Metabolic Syndrome in Kidney Stone Formers: A Comparative Cohort Study with a Median Follow-Up of 19 Years
Reprinted from: *J. Clin. Med.* **2021**, *10*, 978, doi:10.3390/jcm10050978 . . . . **67**

Paul Spiesecke, Thomas Fischer, Frank Friedersdorff, Bernd Hamm and Markus Herbert Lerchbaumer
Quality Assessment of CEUS in Individuals with Small Renal Masses—Which Individual Factors Are Associated with High Image Quality?
Reprinted from: *J. Clin. Med.* **2020**, *9*, 4081, doi:10.3390/jcm9124081 . . . . **77**

Ching-Chia Li, Tsu-Ming Chien, Shu-Pin Huang, Hsin-Chih Yeh, Hsiang-Ying Lee, Hung-Lung Ke, Sheng-Chen Wen, Wei-Che Chang, Yung-Shun Juan, Yii-Her Chou and Wen-Jeng Wu
Single-Site Sutureless Partial Nephrectomy for Small Exophytic Renal Tumors
Reprinted from: *J. Clin. Med.* **2020**, *9*, 3658, doi:10.3390/jcm9113658 . . . . **89**

Francesca J. New, Sally J. Deverill and Bhaskar K. Somani
Outcomes Related to Percutaneous Nephrostomies (PCN) in Malignancy-Associated Ureteric Obstruction: A Systematic Review of the Literature
Reprinted from: *J. Clin. Med.* **2021**, *10*, 2354, doi:10.3390/jcm10112354 . . . . **99**

B. M. Zeeshan Hameed, Aiswarya Dhavileswarapu V. L. S., Syed Zahid Raza, Hadis Karimi, Harneet Singh Khanuja, Dasharathraj K. Shetty, Sufyan Ibrahim, Milap J. Shah, Nithesh Naik, Rahul Paul, Bhavan Prasad Rai and Bhaskar K. Somani
Artificial Intelligence and Its Impact on Urological Diseases and Management: A Comprehensive Review of the Literature
Reprinted from: *J. Clin. Med.* **2021**, *10*, 1864, doi:10.3390/jcm10091864 . . . . **113**

About the Editor

Bhaskar Somani is a Professor of Urology and a Consultant Endourologist at University Hospital Southampton. He has been involved in clinically innovative patient-centred treatments. His research includes minimally invasive surgical techniques (MIST) in management of kidney stone disease and BPH, urinary tract infections, role of mobile phone apps and artificial intelligence (AI) in urology. He is the Clinical Director of 'South Coast Lithotripter Services'. Over the last 10 years his clinical and research work has been covered by BBC, ITV, Daily Mail, The Telegraph and other newspapers and media articles on a number of occasions. He has raised awareness in highlighting risk factors for development of kidney stones such as dehydration, diet and obesity.

He has been a member of BAUS Academic and Endourology sub-sections and is the Wessex Clinical Research Network and Simulation Lead for Urology. He is also the founding member and President of PETRA (Progress in Endourology, Technology and Research Association) Urogroup and i-TRUE (International training and research in uro-oncology and endourology) group, an active member of European School of Urology (ESU) Training and Research group and EAU section of uro-technology (ESUT) endourology group, besides being in the EAU Live surgery and undergraduate training committees.

He is the chosen representative for UK in the Endourology society and in the TOWER research team. He was the advisor to NICE Interventional committee and 'invited expert' to NICE Urological infection guidelines. He coordinates the largest hands-on-training simulation course for urology in the world (EAU-EUREP). He has published over 420 scientific papers, 10 book chapters and has been invited as a speaker, to perform live surgery and for moderations in more than 30 countries worldwide. He has raised a grant income of £3.2million and is in the editorial board of 5 journals. Bhaskar is the course director of UROGRIPP (Urology Global Residents i-TRUE Postgraduate Programme), a modular on-line monthly urology teaching programme attended by 200–500 residents worldwide.

For his work he got awarded the fellowship of Royal College of Edinburgh (Fellow of faculty of Surgical Trainers) in 2017, Honorary Fellowship of Royal College of Physicians and Surgeons of Glasgow in 2020, Endourology Society 'Arthur Smith' award in 2020 and BAUS 'Golden Telescope' and 'Zenith Global' award in 2021. With dedication, commitment and passion for research and teaching, he collaborates nationally and internationally sharing his research and teaching successfully across the world. He has published excellent clinical outcomes and his outcome and research translate into patient benefit.

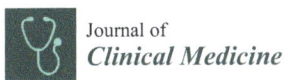

Editorial

Special Issue 'Minimally Invasive Urological Procedures and Related Technological Developments'

Bhaskar Somani

Department of Urology, University Hospital Southampton NHS Trust, Southampton SO16 6YD, UK; bhaskarsomani@yahoo.com

Keywords: kidney calculi; ureteroscopy; PCNL; renal tumour; AI; laser; TFL; urosepsis

The landscape of minimally invasive urological intervention is changing. A great number of new innovations and technological developments have happened over the last three decades, and this is reflected in the publication trends in Urology [1,2]. To address this topic, this Special Issue in the *Journal of Clinical Medicine (JCM)* is dedicated to collecting high-quality scientific contributions focusing mainly on technological developments in managing patients with small renal masses and kidney stone disease.

Two studies investigated the management of small renal masses [3,4]. The first study aimed to identify individual factors in ultrasound (US) that influence contrast-enhanced US (CEUS) image quality, to optimize further imaging workups of incidentally detected focal renal masses. Their findings showed that the focal image quality of CEUS examinations was impaired by a shrunken kidney, a large distance between the kidney and lesion from the body surface, and a smaller lesion size, while the exophytic growth of a focal renal lesion resulted in a better image quality. Awareness of these factors would allow for better patient selection and improve diagnostic confidence in CEUS. In the second study, the authors look at the role of single-site sutureless partial nephrectomy (PN) for small exophytic renal tumors [4]. Of the 52 patients who had laparoscopic PN (LPN), single-site sutureless LPN and traditional suture methods were performed in 33 and 19 patients, respectively. The warm ischemia time and the procedural time were significantly shorter in the sutureless group, showing that it is feasible with small exophytic renal cancer, with excellent cosmetic results and without compromising oncological results.

Several interesting findings were derived from the collective body of work on kidney stone disease (KSD). First, a comparison of holmium low 20W and high 60W Moses laser lithotripsy for ureteroscopy and laser fragmentation (URSL) for KSD was conducted [5]. The use of Moses high-power technology was significantly faster for lithotripsy and significantly reduced the operative time of the second procedure for patients to achieve a stone-free status, with the authors suggesting that a mid-power Moses technology laser was likely to set a new benchmark for treating complex stones, without needing a secondary procedure in most patients. With the advent of the Thulium fiber laser (TFL), the authors of another paper compared the risk of laser fiber fracture between the Ho:YAG laser and TFL with different laser fiber diameters, laser settings, and fibre-bending radii [6]. The authors bench-tested different lengths and radii of the 30WHo:YAG laser and a 50W Super Pulsed TFL, concluding that TFL appeared to be a safer laser with regard to the risk of fiber fracture when used in a deflected position.

Kidney stones are linked to metabolic syndrome (MetS) [7]. In one of the largest comparative cohort studies over a 19-year median follow-up, including 828 stone formers (SF) and 2484 age- and sex-matched non-SF, kidney stone formers were at an increased risk of developing MetS [8]. As stone disease is influenced by dehydration and warm weather [9], in the next paper, the authors looked at global variations in the mineral content of bottled still and sparkling water [10]. In this internationally collaborative study, they

Citation: Somani, B. Special Issue 'Minimally Invasive Urological Procedures and Related Technological Developments'. *J. Clin. Med.* **2021**, *10*, 4225. https://doi.org/10.3390/jcm10184225

Received: 7 September 2021
Accepted: 13 September 2021
Published: 17 September 2021

Publisher's Note: MDPI stays neutral with regard to jurisdictional claims in published maps and institutional affiliations.

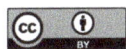

Copyright: © 2021 by the author. Licensee MDPI, Basel, Switzerland. This article is an open access article distributed under the terms and conditions of the Creative Commons Attribution (CC BY) license (https://creativecommons.org/licenses/by/4.0/).

included 316 different still water brands and 224 different sparkling water brands. The authors conclude that as the mineral content of bottled drinking water varies enormously worldwide and as mineral intake through water might influence stone formation, bone health and CVD risk, urologists and nephrologists should counsel their patients on an individual level regarding water intake. The next paper on intervention for KSD looked at the incidence of acute kidney injury (AKI) post percutaneous nephrolithotomy (PNL) in a prospective observational study [11]. Of the 509 patients included, 47 (9.23%) developed postoperative AKI. A higher incidence of AKI was seen in older patients, with associated hypertension and diabetes mellitus, in those receiving ACE inhibitors with lower preoperative hemoglobin and higher serum uric acid, higher stone volume and density, multiple punctures and longer operative time. Patients with AKI also had an increased length of hospital stay, and 17% patients progressed to chronic kidney disease (CKD). The cut-off values for post-PNL AKI were patient age (39.5 years), serum uric acid (4.05 mg/dL) and stone volume (673.06 mm^3). The paper highlights that the strong predictors of post-PNL AKI allow for early identification, proper counseling and postoperative planning and management, in an attempt to avoid further insult to the kidney.

Kidney drainage with percutaneous nephrostomy (PCN) is important in patients with advanced malignancies [12]. This was shown by the authors in their systematic review using 21 full-text articles including 1674 patients. PCN was performed for ureteric obstruction secondary to urological malignancies (37.8%), gynaecological malignancies (26.1%), colorectal and GI malignancies (12.9%), and other specified malignancies (12.2%). The average survival time post-PCN was 5.6 months and varied from 2 to 8.5 months across studies depending on the cancer type, stage and previous treatment. Their results showed that patients with advanced malignancies who needed PCN tended to have a survival rate under 12 months and spend a large proportion of this time in the hospital. They concluded that decisions about PCN must be balanced with survival and quality of life, which must be discussed with the patient. While extracorporeal shock wave lithotripsy (ESWL) treatment is used for KSD, in the next paper, the authors used extracorporeal shockwave therapy (ESWT) in patients with chronic prostatitis/chronic pelvic pain syndrome (CP/CPPS) [13]. From this perspective, a single-arm cohort study of a total of 215 patients, with an established diagnosis of CP/CPPS, underwent perineal ESWT once a week for six consecutive weeks with a protocol of 3000 pulses at an energy of 0.25 mJoule/mm^2 and a frequency of 4 Hertz (Hz). Over 12 months, this study showed that ESWT was an outpatient, easy-to-perform, and minimally invasive procedure, alleviating pain and improving erectile function and quality of life in patients with refractory CP/CPPS.

Finally, the last two papers looked at the role of artificial intelligence (AI), which has quickly been growing in the field of urology [14–16]. The first paper looked at the role and impact of AI on urological diseases in a large comprehensive review of literature [15]. It covers the usage of AI in prostate cancer, urothelial cancer, renal cancer, reflux disease, reproductive urology, urolithiasis, paediatric urology and other endourological procedures. Furthermore, the role it plays in renal transplant, radiotherapy and robotic surgery is also covered in detail. The second paper on AI looked at a machine learning (ML) predictive model for post-ureteroscopy urosepsis in patients who needed intensive care unit (ICU) admission [16]. In this retrospective case–control study, the risk factors for urosepsis were predicted with reasonable accuracy by their innovative ML model. The authors conclude that focusing on these risk factors will allow clinicians to create predictive strategies to minimize post-operative morbidity.

Several interesting findings are derived from this collective body of work. While technological advances were addressed in combatting small renal masses and kidney stone disease, newer tools for diagnostic and surgical interventions were also covered. There are still many fundamental questions that need more evidence in order to be answered, relating to cost and quality of life management for these patients [17,18]. As the Guest Editor, I would like to give special thanks to the reviewers for their professional comments and to the *JCM* team for their robust support. Finally, I sincerely thank all the authors for their valuable contributions.

Funding: This research received no external funding.

Conflicts of Interest: The author declares no conflict of interest.

References

1. Pietropaolo, A.; Proietti, S.; Geraghty, R.; Skolarikos, A.; Papatsoris, A.; Liatsikos, E.; Somani, B.K. Trends of 'urolithiasis: Interventions, simulation, and laser technology' over the last 16 years (2000–2015) as published in the literature (PubMed): A systematic review from European section of Uro-technology (ESUT). *World J. Urol.* **2017**, *35*, 1651–1658. [CrossRef] [PubMed]
2. Geraghty, R.M.; Jones, P.; Somani, B. Worldwide Trends of Urinary Stone Disease Treatment Over the Last Two Decades: A Systematic Review. *J. Endourol.* **2017**, *31*, 547–556. [CrossRef] [PubMed]
3. Spiesecke, P.; Fischer, T.; Friedersdorff, F.; Hamm, B.; Lerchbaumer, M.H. Quality Assessment of CEUS in Individuals with Small Renal Masses—Which Individual Factors Are Associated with High Image Quality? *J. Clin. Med.* **2020**, *9*, 4081. [CrossRef]
4. Li, C.-C.; Chien, T.-M.; Huang, S.-P.; Yeh, H.-C.; Lee, H.-Y.; Ke, H.-L.; Wen, S.-C.; Chang, W.-C.; Juan, Y.-S.; Chou, Y.-H.; et al. Single-Site Sutureless Partial Nephrectomy for Small Exophytic Renal Tumors. *J. Clin. Med.* **2020**, *9*, 3658. [CrossRef] [PubMed]
5. Pietropaolo, A.; Hughes, T.; Mani, M.; Somani, B. Outcomes of Ureteroscopy and Laser Stone Fragmentation (URSL) for Kidney Stone Disease (KSD): Comparative Cohort Study Using MOSES Technology 60 W Laser System versus Regular Holmium 20 W Laser. *J. Clin. Med.* **2021**, *10*, 2742. [CrossRef] [PubMed]
6. Uzan, A.; Chiron, P.; Panthier, F.; Haddad, M.; Berthe, L.; Traxer, O.; Doizi, S. Comparison of Holmium:YAG and Thulium Fiber Lasers on the Risk of Laser Fiber Fracture. *J. Clin. Med.* **2021**, *10*, 2960. [CrossRef] [PubMed]
7. Wong, Y.V.; Cook, P.; Somani, B.K. The Association of Metabolic Syndrome and Urolithiasis. *Int. J. Endocrinol.* **2015**, *2015*, 1–9. [CrossRef] [PubMed]
8. Geraghty, R.; Cook, P.; Roderick, P.; Somani, B. Risk of Metabolic Syndrome in Kidney Stone Formers: A Comparative Cohort Study with a Median Follow-Up of 19 Years. *J. Clin. Med.* **2021**, *10*, 978. [CrossRef] [PubMed]
9. Geraghty, R.M.; Proietti, S.; Traxer, O.; Archer, M.; Somani, B.K. Worldwide Impact of Warmer Seasons on the Incidence of Renal Colic and Kidney Stone Disease: Evidence from a Systematic Review of Literature. *J. Endourol.* **2017**, *31*, 729–735. [CrossRef] [PubMed]
10. Stoots, S.; Kamphuis, G.; Geraghty, R.; Vogt, L.; Henderickx, M.; Hameed, B.; Ibrahim, S.; Pietropaolo, A.; Jamnadass, E.; Aljumaiah, S.; et al. Global Variations in the Mineral Content of Bottled Still and Sparkling Water and a Description of the Possible Impact on Nephrological and Urological Diseases. *J. Clin. Med.* **2021**, *10*, 2807. [CrossRef] [PubMed]
11. Pillai, S.; Kriplani, A.; Chawla, A.; Somani, B.; Pandey, A.; Prabhu, R.; Choudhury, A.; Pandit, S.; Taori, R.; Hegde, P. Acute Kidney Injury Post-Percutaneous Nephrolithotomy (PNL): Prospective Outcomes from a University Teaching Hospital. *J. Clin. Med.* **2021**, *10*, 1373. [CrossRef]
12. New, F.; Deverill, S.; Somani, B. Outcomes Related to Percutaneous Nephrostomies (PCN) in Malignancy-Associated Ureteric Obstruction: A Systematic Review of the Literature. *J. Clin. Med.* **2021**, *10*, 2354. [CrossRef]
13. Wu, W.-L.; Bamodu, O.A.; Wang, Y.-H.; Hu, S.-W.; Tzou, K.-Y.; Yeh, C.-T.; Wu, C.-C. Extracorporeal Shockwave Therapy (ESWT) Alleviates Pain, Enhances Erectile Function and Improves Quality of Life in Patients with Chronic Prostatitis/Chronic Pelvic Pain Syndrome. *J. Clin. Med.* **2021**, *10*, 3602. [CrossRef] [PubMed]
14. Shah, M.; Naik, N.; Somani, B.K.; Hameed, B.M.Z. Artificial intelligence (AI) in urology-Current use and future directions: An iTRUE study. *Türk Üroloji Dergisi/Turkish J. Urol.* **2020**, *46*, S27–S39. [CrossRef] [PubMed]
15. Hameed, B.; Dhavileswarapu, A.S.; Raza, S.; Karimi, H.; Khanuja, H.; Shetty, D.; Ibrahim, S.; Shah, M.; Naik, N.; Paul, R.; et al. Artificial Intelligence and Its Impact on Urological Diseases and Management: A Comprehensive Review of the Literature. *J. Clin. Med.* **2021**, *10*, 1864. [CrossRef] [PubMed]
16. Pietropaolo, A.; Geraghty, R.M.; Veeratterapillay, R.; Rogers, A.; Kallidonis, P.; Villa, L.; Boeri, L.; Montanari, E.; Atis, G.; Emiliani, E.; et al. A Machine Learning Predictive Model for Post-Ureteroscopy Urosepsis Needing Intensive Care Unit Admission: A Case–Control YAU Endourology Study from Nine European Centres. *J. Clin. Med.* **2021**, *10*, 3888. [CrossRef] [PubMed]
17. Somani, B.K.; Robertson, A.; Kata, S.G. Decreasing the Cost of Flexible Ureterorenoscopic Procedures. *Urology* **2011**, *78*, 528–530. [CrossRef] [PubMed]
18. Jones, P.; Pietropaolo, A.; Chew, B.H.; Somani, B.K. Atlas of scoring systems, grading tools and nomograms in Endourology: A comprehensive overview from The TOWER Endourological Society research group. *J. Endourol.* **2021**. [CrossRef]

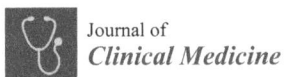

Article

A Machine Learning Predictive Model for Post-Ureteroscopy Urosepsis Needing Intensive Care Unit Admission: A Case–Control YAU Endourology Study from Nine European Centres

Amelia Pietropaolo [1], Robert M. Geraghty [2], Rajan Veeratterapillay [2], Alistair Rogers [2], Panagiotis Kallidonis [3], Luca Villa [4], Luca Boeri [5], Emanuele Montanari [5], Gokhan Atis [6], Esteban Emiliani [7], Tarik Emre Sener [8], Feras Al Jaafari [9], John Fitzpatrick [2], Matthew Shaw [2], Chris Harding [2] and Bhaskar K. Somani [1,*]

1. Department of Urology, University Hospital Southampton, Southampton SO16 6YD, UK; ameliapietr@gmail.com
2. Department of Urology, Freeman Hospital, Freeman Road, Newcastle-upon-Tyne NE1 7DN, UK; robgeraghty@btinternet.com (R.M.G.); r.veeratterapillay@nhs.net (R.V.); Alistair.rogers2@nhs.net (A.R.); john.fitzpatrick4@nhs.net (J.F.); Matthew.shaw7@nhs.net (M.S.); c.harding@nhs.net (C.H.)
3. Department of Urology, University of Patras, 26504 Patras, Greece; pkallidonis@yahoo.com
4. IRCCS Ospedale San Raffaele, Urology, 20019 Milan, Italy; lucavilla01984@gmail.com
5. Department of Urology, IRCCS Fondazione Ca' Granda-Ospedale Maggiore Policlinico, University of Milan, 20019 Milan, Italy; dr.lucaboeri@gmail.com (L.B.); montanari.emanuele@gmail.com (E.M.)
6. Department of Urology, Faculty of Medicine, Istanbul Medeniyet University, Istanbul 34720, Turkey; gokhanatis@hotmail.com
7. Department of Urology, Fundació Puigvert, 08001 Barcelona, Spain; emiliani@gmail.com
8. Department of Urology, Marmara University, Istanbul 34720, Turkey; dr.emresener@gmail.com
9. Victoria Hospital, Kirkcaldy KY1 2ND, UK; feras.al.jaafari@gmail.com
* Correspondence: bhaskarsomani@yahoo.com; Tel.: +44-23-8120-6873

Abstract: Introduction: With the rise in the use of ureteroscopy and laser stone lithotripsy (URSL), a proportionate increase in the risk of post-procedural urosepsis has also been observed. The aims of our paper were to analyse the predictors for severe urosepsis using a machine learning model (ML) in patients that needed intensive care unit (ICU) admission and to make comparisons with a matched cohort. Methods: A retrospective study was conducted across nine high-volume endourology European centres for all patients who underwent URSL and subsequently needed ICU admission for urosepsis (Group A). This was matched by patients with URSL without urosepsis (Group B). Statistical analysis was performed with 'R statistical software' using the 'randomforests' package. The data were segregated at random into a 70% training set and a 30% test set using the 'sample' command. A random forests ML model was then built with $n = 300$ trees, with the test set used for internal validation. Diagnostic accuracy statistics were generated using the 'caret' package. Results: A total of 114 patients were included (57 in each group) with a mean age of 60 ± 16 years and a male:female ratio of 1:1.19. The ML model correctly predicted risk of sepsis in 14/17 (82%) cases (Group A) and predicted those without urosepsis for 12/15 (80%) controls (Group B), whilst overall it also discriminated between the two groups predicting both those with and without sepsis. Our model accuracy was 81.3% (95%, CI: 63.7–92.8%), sensitivity = 0.80, specificity = 0.82 and area under the curve = 0.89. Predictive values most commonly accounting for nodal points in the trees were a large proximal stone location, long stent time, large stone size and long operative time. Conclusion: Urosepsis after endourological procedures remains one of the main reasons for ICU admission. Risk factors for urosepsis are reasonably accurately predicted by our innovative ML model. Focusing on these risk factors can allow one to create predictive strategies to minimise post-operative morbidity.

Keywords: kidney stones; urosepsis; ureteroscopy; laser lithotripsy; urolithiasis; nephrolithiasis; kidney calculi; predictor factors

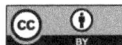

1. Introduction

Kidney stones disease (KSD) has seen an increase in incidence and prevalence over the last few decades [1–4]. This can vary according to the ethnicity, geographical origin and weather along with diet and behavioural variations such as exercise, diet and fluid intake [2,3]. Treatment options consist of shockwave lithotripsy (SWL), ureteroscopy and laser stone lithotripsy (URSL) and percutaneous nephrolithotomy (PCNL) in accordance with the stone size and location [2,3].

URSL is becoming an increasingly common procedure to treat kidney and ureteral stones. There has been an upwards trend of URSL over the last few years, becoming a popular surgical procedure for KSD [4]. Despite being minimally invasive in nature, the use of high-pressure irrigation and the dispersion of potential infected stone particles can cause urinary tract infections (UTIs), and, in rare cases, it can cause severe systemic infection and sepsis. Post-ureteroscopic infectious complications and urosepsis are uncommon but serious life-threatening complications and range from 2.2% to 20% in several studies [5]. They affect the immunological system but also coagulation, the central nervous system, the autonomic nervous system, the endocrine system, the cardiovascular system, the liver and the kidneys [6].

The term systemic inflammatory response syndrome (SIRS) has been previously used along with the term severe sepsis and septic shock. While the SIRS criteria include fever, tachycardia, tachypnoea and raised serum inflammatory markers, having two or more of these is called sepsis. The sequential organ failure assessment (SOFA) score, which is an index of organ dysfunction secondary to infection, was used to predict ICU mortality based on laboratory results and clinical data. High SOFA score immediately correlates to the risk of mortality [7]. The predictive value of the SOFA score for in-hospital mortality was superior to that of the SIRS criteria. The Third International Consensus Definitions for 'Sepsis and Septic Shock' (sepsis 3) updated the definition of sepsis [8]. The presence of >2 criteria were identified under quick SOFA (qSOFA) score.

Sepsis can also present as septic shock characterised by severe cardio-circulatory compromise, requiring multiorgan support, adequate fluid resuscitation and intensive care unit (ICU) support [9]. Management of sepsis includes intervention at multiple levels, from administration of antibiotics to fluid resuscitation, hemofiltration, cardiovascular and respiratory support. Furthermore, the long-term social, physical, psychological and cognitive disabilities of patients who survive sepsis require huge healthcare and social support with consequent economic impact [10].

Severe urosepsis can lead to multiorgan failure and death. Mortality secondary to ureteroscopy has risen over the past decade. In a recent systematic review, the cause of death after URSL for stone disease was found to be sepsis in over half of all reported patients [11]. The aim of our paper was to analyse the predictors for severe urosepsis in patients that needed ICU admission. We used a matched ureteroscopy cohort, with which we built a machine learning (ML) model to predict which patients would develop urosepsis needing ICU treatment.

2. Methods

A retrospective study was conducted across 9 high-volume endourology European centres from 5 countries (Italy, Greece, Turkey, Spain and the UK). The inclusion criteria were all patients who underwent URSL for stone disease and subsequently developed urosepsis that needed ICU admission (Group A). This was matched by a similar group of patients who had a URSL procedure for stone disease without urosepsis (Group B). The data on patient demographics, comorbidities, ASA grade, previous history of UTIs, prior endoscopic procedures, pre-operative urine culture and laboratory parameters for infection both pre- and post-surgery were collected over an 11-year period from these centres between 2009 and 2020.

While the study included patients who developed urosepsis that needed ICU admission, patients with non-infectious complications and not needing ICU were excluded.

Urinary tract infection was defined as a positive urine culture with >10⁴ colony forming units per millilitre (CFU)/mL. Information on empirical and selective antibiotics used was also collected. Further variables were analysed with particular attention towards stent dwell time, intraoperative use of ureteral access sheath (UAS) and operative time. Primary and secondary outcomes were complication and stone-free rates (SFR), respectively. Cases were matched with the control group (Group B) for age; gender; and comorbidities known to increase the risk of post-ureteroscopic UTI: diabetes mellitus (DM), immunosuppression, neurological disorders, previous urinary tract reconstruction and abnormal upper tract anatomy [12].

Statistical analysis was performed using R (R statistical software, Vienna, Austria) using the 'randomforests' package. The data were segregated at random into a 70% training set and a 30% test set using the 'sample' command with the seed set at 1234. A random forests machine learning model was then built with $n = 300$ trees, with the test set used for internal validation. A random forests model generates a set number (i.e., 300 in this case) of random decision trees, which are then aggregated to form the single model. Diagnostic accuracy statistics (sensitivity, specificity and area under the curve) for model performance were generated using the 'caret' package. Graphs were generated using 'ggplot2', and these include a receiver operator curve (ROC) for the model, along with a 'mean decrease gini' plot (demonstrates variables ranked according to how frequently they are represented in the random trees prior to aggregation—more important variables will be represented more frequently). Explanatory graphs with individual predictions are presented following generation with the 'lime' (local interpretable model agnostic explanations) package. The model was deployed as a 'shiny' application using the 'shiny' package.

3. Results

A total of 114 patients were included (57 in each group) with a mean age of 60 years (±16) with a male:female ratio of 1:1.19 in both groups (Table 1).

The numbers of patients in Groups A and B with DM ($n = 15$, 26.3% and $n = 12$, 21.1%), immunocompromise ($n = 3$ and 1), neurological disorder ($n = 1$ and 1), previous urinary tract reconstruction ($n = 1$ and 0) and abnormal upper tract anatomy ($n = 1$ and 5) were as shown. There were 14 (24.6%) and 3 (5.3%) patients with a history of UTI for Groups A and B, respectively. Indwelling stent dwell time for Groups A and B were 52 ± 63 days and 30 ± 60 days for 33 and 26 patients, respectively. In each group, 31 patients (54.3%) had a single stone; the remaining (45.6%) had more than one stone (range: 2–5). The single largest stone sizes in Groups A and B were 10 ± 5 mm and 8 ± 4 mm, respectively. In both groups, 15 patients (26.3%) had a pre-operative positive urine culture that was treated as per local protocol. The mean operative time was 58 ± 31 min and 43 ± 23 min, and the SFR was 48.6% and 89.5% in Groups A and B, respectively. One patient in Group A (83-year-old female) died from urosepsis. She also had a history of prior recurrent UTIs, was ASA 3 and suffered with Alzheimer's dementia. She was not pre-stented, no access sheath was used, and a procedural time of 45 min with a post-operative stent left in situ was noted. She developed multi-resistant *Escherichia coli* infection and died of septic shock after 2 days.

Table 1. Patient characteristics of both Groups A and B.

		Group A, n = 57	Group B, n = 57
Mean age (years) ± SD		60 ± 16	60 ± 16
Male gender, n (%)		26 (45.6%)	26 (45.6%)
Diabetes, n (%)		15 (26.3%)	12 (21.1%)
Immunosuppression/modulation, n (%)		3 (5.3%)	1 (1.8%)
Neurological disorder, n (%)		1 (1.8%)	1 (1.8%)
Previous urinary tract reconstruction, n (%)		1 (1.8%)	0
Abnormal upper tract anatomy, n (%)		1 (1.8%)	5 (8.8%)
History of recurrent UTI, n (%)		14 (24.6%)	3 (5.3%)
Emergency admission		30 (52.6%)	9 (15.8%)
Presence of pre-operative stent, n (%)		33 (57.9%)	26 (45.6%)
Mean stent dwell time (days) ± SD		52 ± 63	30 ± 60
Number of stones	1	31	31
	2	20	13
	3	3	13
	4	2	0
	5	1	0
Mean largest stone diameter (mm) ± SD		10 ± 5	8 ± 4
Location, n	Vesicoureteric junction (VUJ)	3	3
	Distal ureter	7	11
	Mid ureter	8	11
	Proximal ureter	8	13
	Renal	31	15
	N/A	0	4
Positive pre-operative urine culture, n (%)		15 (26.3%)	15 (26.3%)
Mean operative time (mins) ± SD		58 ± 31	43 ± 23
Post-operative stent insertion, n (%)		36 (46.2%)	42 (53.8%)
Stone free, n (%)		34 (48.6%)	51 (89.5%)

The ML model correctly predicted risk of sepsis in 14/17 (82%) cases (Group A) and predicted those without urosepsis for 12/15 (80%) controls (Group B), whilst, overall, it also discriminated between the two groups, predicting both those with and without sepsis. Our model accuracy was 81.3% (95%, CI: 63.7–92.8%), sensitivity = 0.80, specificity = 0.82 and area under the curve = 0.89. Predictive values most commonly accounting for nodal points in the trees were large proximal stone location, long stent time, large stone size and long operative time (Figures 1 and 2). The model was deployed onto the internet using the 'shiny' application. Users are able to input patient, stone and operative characteristics for an outcome prediction. The outcome prediction is either 'sepsis' or 'no sepsis' and is presented using the 'lime' package, which demonstrates which variables are affecting the outcome most within the context of the model (see Figure 3 and https://endourology.shinyapps.io/Urosepsis_Predictor/, accessed on 22 August 2021).

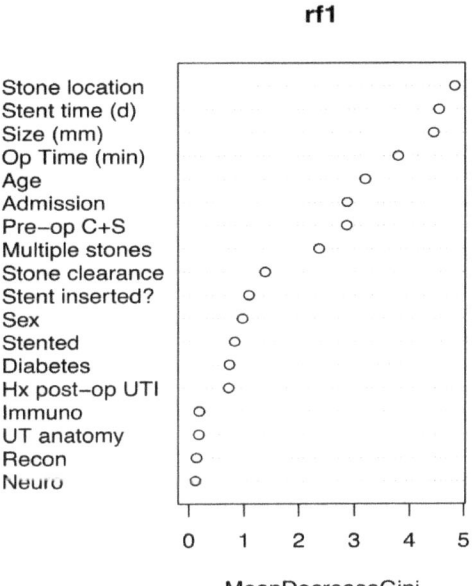

Figure 1. Gini is a graph of factors most commonly represented in the random trees ($n = 300$ trees) produced prior to tree aggregation to form the model. The more frequently the variable is represented, the more important the variable will be to the final model.

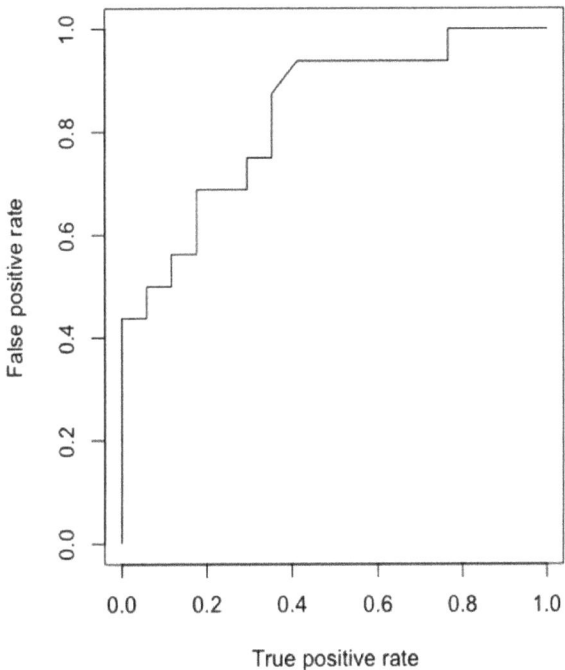

Figure 2. Receiver operator curve (ROC) for internally validated model.

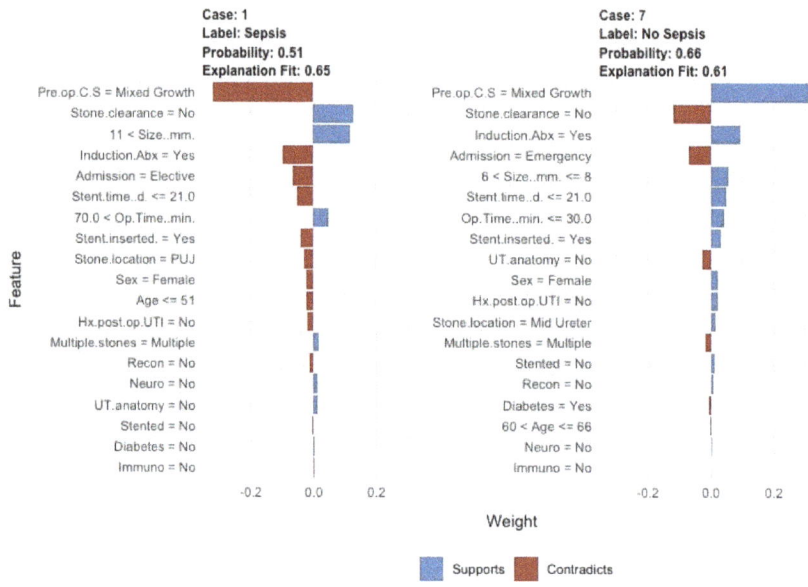

Figure 3. Lime (local interpretable model-agnostic explanations graphs) deployed for the model. Predictions are given on a case-by-case basis, along with the explanatory variables contributing to that outcome, within the context of the model.

4. Discussion

4.1. Meaning of the Study

In the current study, we used data collected from different centres across Europe to develop an easy-to-use machine learning tool for prediction of post-operative sepsis and ICU admission in patients undergoing elective URSL for stone disease. Using a machine-learning approach, we found that proximal stone location, long stent dwelling time, large stone size and long operative time can reasonably accurately identify patients at risk of developing post-operative urosepsis.

All predictive parameters analysed in our model are part of the routine assessment to identify the indication for surgery, and this makes our model accessible to all urologists. Preoperative identification of those patients who have a higher risk of developing sepsis or requiring post-operative ICU can help to create preventative strategies such as focusing on antibiotic prophylaxis, preoperative counselling and intraoperative support. This may also prevent exposure of low-risk patients to unnecessary antibiotic therapy.

4.2. Risk Factors of Post-Ureteroscopic Urosepsis from Previous Published Literature

This topic has been the subject of heated debate in the last few years, with many published studies attempting to identify common risk factors of post-operative urosepsis. However, no other studies to date have used a machine learning model to predict risk factors of urosepsis. A recent study by Bhanot et al. identified urosepsis with a higher risk of death after URSL procedures [11]. Predictors identified in their systematic review allowed the creation of recommendations, such as preoperative urine culture and appropriate treatment; reducing the operative time; trying to favour staged procedures, especially in patients with large stone burden; and minimising stent dwell time. Care in preoperative assessment and postoperative monitoring was identified as a strategy for early detection of complications and minimising the risk of mortality.

A recent study demonstrated individual risk factors for urosepsis [12]. Chugh et al. carried out a systematic review of the literature to identify predictors of infectious complications following URSL for stone disease. Patients with multiple comorbidities, such as obesity, old age, female gender, neurogenic bladder, long operative time and indwelling ureteric stents, were shown to be related to a higher risk for UTIs or sepsis. Strategies such as prophylactic antibiotics, limiting stent dwell or procedural time and staging procedures were identified as possible preventative measures. Similar parameters were identified by Southern et al. [13], who retrospectively analysed 3298 patients undergoing URSL for stone disease and found that 7% of them developed post-operative SIRS/febrile UTIs. In their multivariate logistic regression, the authors found that female gender, surgical time and positive preoperative urine culture were predictors for infectious complications.

Prior emergency decompression for infected obstructed kidney may appear as a possible risk factor for urosepsis. However, in a study by Pietropaolo et al., only 1.2% developed sepsis after elective stone removal in such patients [14], demonstrating that initial septic presentation is not a risk factor for post-operative urosepsis when it comes to elective URSL. Martov et al., on behalf of CROES group [15], collected data from 1325 patients who underwent URSL for renal and ureteric stones. They identified predictive factors of postoperative UTI and fever as female gender, Crohn's disease, cardiovascular disease, high stone burden and an ASA score of 2 or higher.

A Chinese group in a study conducted by Xu et al. [16] studied the trend of the serum parameter bone morphogenetic protein endothelial cell precursor-derived regulator (BMPER) in patients with urosepsis following ureteroscopic stone treatment. They concluded that a high BMPER concentration is a strong predictor of adverse outcome in patients with post-operative urosepsis. In their meta-analysis, Bhojani et al. [17] found six risk factors statistically associated with increased postoperative urosepsis risk, such as preoperative stent, positive preoperative urine culture, ischaemic heart disease, older age, longer procedure time and diabetes mellitus. Bai et al. retrospectively reviewed 1421 patients who underwent ureteroscopy and stone laser treatment and found that patients with positive preoperative urine culture or long operation duration had a higher risk of developing urosepsis after URSL [18].

4.3. Comparison with Other ML Studies

The role of artificial intelligence (AI) in medicine is expanding day-by-day due to its capability of performing human cognitive tasks. The huge amount of data extracted by the electronic medical records can be used for computer-based predictions that can help in improving patient care [19]. There are four subfields of AI in health care, and machine learning (ML) is one of them. This is a technique that uses algorithms and allows a computer to recognise patterns and learn automatically through experience and by the use of data. The method is being increasingly used in all medical specialties, including urology, and its use is already widespread in all urological subspecialties. Song et al. [20] in their review assessed whether ML models were superior compared to logistic regression (LR), a more conventional prediction model. They used both techniques in predicting acute kidney injury (AKI) and agreed that in the literature, ML was superior due to its more variable and adaptable performance.

Aminsharifi et al. [21] analysed data of 146 adult patients who underwent percutaneous nephrolithotomy (PCNL) to validate the efficiency of an ML algorithm for predicting the outcomes after PCNL. This program predicted the PCNL results with an accuracy of up to 95%. Blum et al. [22] created an ML framework to improve the early detection of clinically significant hydronephrosis caused by pelvic–ureteric junction obstruction based on data from renograms. This had a 93% accuracy in predicting earlier detection of severe cases requiring surgery.

ML is also utilised in cancer diagnosis or treatment outcomes. Kocak et al. [23] developed models for distinguishing three major subtypes of renal cell carcinomas (RCC) using an ML model based on CT scan results. The model could satisfactorily distinguish non-RCC from RCC. Similarly, Feng et al. [24] used a ML approach to accurately discriminate between small angiomyolipoma (AML) and RCC in CT scans with high accuracy, sensitivity and specificity. Hasnain et al. [25] used an ML algorithm to predict cancer recurrence and survival after radical cystectomy based on imaging, operative findings and pathology. Deng et al. [26] developed an ML algorithm that could differentiate metastatic castrate-resistant prostate cancer patients in two groups, those who could tolerate docetaxel and those who could not. This model managed to predict therapeutic failure in patients who could potentially develop toxic effects of docetaxel chemotherapy.

4.4. Strengths, Limitations and Areas of Future Research

The machine learning models provide a new benchmark for predicting surgical or oncological outcomes and highlight opportunities for improving care using optimal preoperative and operative data collection. The limitation of our study is based on its retrospective nature. Further prospective and randomised controlled trials are required to corroborate our findings and to be able to write specific recommendations that will allow the prediction of post-URSL sepsis. Furthermore, external validation of our ML model is required to confirm its effectiveness and predictive power, with subsequent development of a mobile-phone app to be used in day-to-day clinical practice.

Genetics has recently been introduced as a new field of research on the topic by Giamarellos-Bourboulis et al. [27]. They have related low concentrations of immunoglobulins with adverse outcomes in urosepsis response. Carriage of minor genetic deficiency in antibody production can be related to poor sepsis prognosis. This field has not been fully exploited to date, but a genomic approach should be taken into consideration in the future as an aid to identify the origin of this deadly disease.

Urosepsis requiring ICU support is a rare post-operative event and, despite multiple centres involved in data collection, only few cases were available for analysis. AI and ML models are certainly expected to play an increasing role in the medical field due to the global technological advancement and their capability of learning and reproducing tasks without instructions. However, the topic is complex, and issues exist regarding the reliability of machine diagnosis, the consent for data sharing and the external control of large industries or data holders with the inherent conflict of interest this brings. Nevertheless, future applications of ML models are yet to come, and the use of these algorithms can only increase.

5. Conclusions

Urosepsis after endourological procedures, such as URSL, remains one of the main causes for ICU admission and consequent post-operative disabilities or mortality. Risk factors for urosepsis are reasonably accurately predicted by our innovative machine learning model. Focusing on these risk factors can allow one to create predictive strategies to minimise post-operative morbidity. External validation of the model is required to confirm its effectiveness in predicting sepsis.

Author Contributions: Study design/concept: A.P. and B.K.S.; data collection: A.P., R.M.G., R.V., A.R., P.K., L.V., L.B., G.A., E.E., T.E.S. and F.A.J.; data analysis: R.M.G.; manuscript draft: A.P.; critical appraisal of manuscript: E.M., J.F., M.S., C.H. and B.K.S. All authors have read and agreed to the published version of the manuscript.

Funding: No funding was received for this paper.

Institutional Review Board Statement: The study was conducted according to the guidelines of the Declaration of Helsinki, and approved by the Ethics Committee of University of Southampton (protocol code 6212 on 1/3/2021).

Informed Consent Statement: Informed consent was obtained from all subjects involved in the study.

Data Availability Statement: As data is identifiable, it will not be made available as per ethical approval.

Acknowledgments: We would like to thank all of the hospitals and surgeons for contributing data.

Conflicts of Interest: No conflict of interest.

References

1. Geraghty, R.M.; Proietti, S.; Traxer, O.; Archer, M.; Somani, B.K. Worldwide impact of warmer seasons on the incidence of renal colic and kidney stone disease: Evidence from a systematic review of literature. *J. Endourol.* **2017**, *31*, 729–735. [CrossRef]
2. Assimos, D.; Krambeck, A.; Miller, N.L.; Monga, M.; Murad, M.H.; Nelson, C.P.; Pace, K.T.; Pais, V.M.; Pearle, M.S.; Preminger, G.M.; et al. Surgical management of stones: American Urological Association/Endourological Society guideline, PART I. *J. Urol.* **2016**, *196*, 1153–1160. [CrossRef]
3. Türk, C.; Neisius, A.; Petřík, A.; Seitz, C.; Skolarikos, A.; Somani, B.; Thomas, K.; Gambaro, G. EAU Guidelines on urolithiasis. *Eur. Assoc. Urol.* **2021**. Available online: https://uroweb.org/guideline/urolithiasis/# (accessed on 22 August 2021).
4. Pietropaolo, A.; Proietti, S.; Geraghty, R.; Skolarikos, A.; Papatsoris, A.; Liatsikos, E.; Somani, B.K. Trends of 'urolithiasis: Interventions, simulation, and laser technology' over the last 16 years (2000–2015) as published in the literature (PubMed): A systematic review from European section of Uro-technology (ESUT). *World J. Urol.* **2017**, *35*, 1651–1658. [CrossRef] [PubMed]
5. Bonkat, G.; Cai, T.; Veeratterapillay, R.; Bruyere, F.; Bartoletti, R.; Pilatz, A.; Köves, B.; Geerlings, S.E.; Pradere, B.; Pickard, R.; et al. Management of Urosepsis in 2018. *Eur. Urol. Focus* **2019**, *5*, 5–9. [CrossRef] [PubMed]
6. Wagenlehner, F.M.; Tandogdu, Z.; Johansen, T.E.B. An update on classification and management of urosepsis. *Curr. Opin. Urol.* **2017**, *27*, 133–137. [CrossRef] [PubMed]
7. Marik, P.E.; Taeb, A.M. SIRS, qSOFA and new sepsis definition. *J. Thorac. Dis.* **2017**, *9*, 943–945. [CrossRef]
8. Singer, M.; Deutschman, C.S.; Seymour, C.W.; Shankar-Hari, M.; Annane, D.; Bauer, M.; Bellomo, R.; Bernard, G.R.; Chiche, J.D.; Coopersmith, C.M.; et al. The Third International Consensus Definitions for Sepsis and Septic Shock (Sepsis-3). *JAMA* **2016**, *315*, 801–810. [CrossRef]
9. Seymour, C.W.; Liu, V.X.; Iwashyna, T.J.; Brunkhorst, F.M.; Rea, T.D.; Scherag, A.; Rubenfeld, G.; Kahn, J.M.; Shankar Hari, M.; Singer, M.; et al. Assessment of clinical criteria for sepsis. *JAMA* **2016**, *315*, 762–774. [CrossRef]
10. Dellinger, R.P.; Levy, M.M.; Rhodes, A.; Annane, D.; Gerlach, H.; Opal, S.M.; Sevransky, J.E.; Sprung, C.L.; Douglas, I.S.; Jaeschke, R.; et al. Surviving sepsis campaign: International guidelines for management of severe sepsis and septic shock: 2012. *Crit. Care Med.* **2013**, *41*, 580–637. [CrossRef]
11. Bhanot, R.; Pietropaolo, A.; Tokas, T.; Kallidonis, P.; Skolarikos, A.; Keller, E.X.; De Coninck, V.; Traxer, O.; Gozen, A.; Sarica, K.; et al. Predictors and Strategies to Avoid Mortality Following Ureteroscopy for Stone Disease: A Systematic Review from European Association of Urologists Sections of Urolithiasis (EULIS) and Uro-technology (ESUT). *Eur. Urol. Focus* **2021**. [CrossRef] [PubMed]
12. Chugh, S.; Pietropaolo, A.; Montanari, E.; Sarica, K.; Somani, B.K. Predictors of Urinary Infections and Urosepsis after Ureteroscopy for Stone Disease: A Systematic Review from EAU Section of Urolithiasis (EULIS). *Curr. Urol. Rep.* **2020**, *21*, 16. [CrossRef]
13. Southern, J.B.; Higgins, A.M.; Young, A.J.; Kost, K.A.; Schreiter, B.R.; Clifton, M.; Fulmer, B.R.; Garg, T. Risk Factors for Postoperative Fever and Systemic Inflammatory Response Syndrome After Ureteroscopy for Stone Disease. *J. Endourol.* **2019**, *33*, 516–522. [CrossRef]
14. Pietropaolo, A.; Hendry, J.; Kyriakides, R.; Geraghty, R.; Jones, P.; Aboumarzouk, O.; Somani, B.K. Outcomes of Elective Ureteroscopy for Ureteric Stones in Patients with Prior Urosepsis and Emergency Drainage: Prospective Study over 5 yr from a Tertiary Endourology Centre. *Eur. Urol. Focus* **2020**, *6*, 151–156. [CrossRef] [PubMed]
15. Martov, A.; Gravas, S.; Etemadian, M.; Unsal, A.; Barusso, G.; D'Addessi, A.; Krambeck, A.; De La Rosette, J.; Clinical Research Office of the Endourological Society Ureteroscopy Study Group. Postoperative infection rates in patients with a negative baseline urine culture undergoing ureteroscopic stone removal: A matched case-control analysis on antibiotic prophylaxis from the CROES URS global study. *J. Endourol.* **2015**, *29*, 171–180. [CrossRef] [PubMed]
16. Xu, C.G.; Guo, Y.L. Diagnostic and Prognostic Values of BMPER in Patients with Urosepsis following Ureteroscopic Lithotripsy. *Biomed. Res. Int.* **2019**, *2019*, 8078139. [CrossRef] [PubMed]
17. Bhojani, N.; Miller, L.E.; Bhattacharyya, S.; Cutone, B.; Chew, B.H. Risk Factors for Urosepsis After Ureteroscopy for Stone Disease: A Systematic Review with Meta-Analysis. *J. Endourol.* **2021**, *35*, 991–1000. [CrossRef]
18. Bai, T.; Yu, X.; Qin, C.; Xu, T.; Shen, H.; Wang, L.; Liu, X. Identification of Factors Associated with Postoperative Urosepsis after Ureteroscopy with Holmium: Yttrium-Aluminum-Garnet Laser Lithotripsy. *Urol. Int.* **2019**, *103*, 311–317. [CrossRef]
19. Shah, M.; Naik, N.; Somani, B.K.; Hameed, B.Z. Artificial intelligence (AI) in urology-Current use and future directions: An iTRUE study. *Turk. J. Urol.* **2020**, *46* (Suppl. 1), S27–S39. [CrossRef]
20. Song, X.; Liu, X.; Liu, F.; Wang, C. Comparison of machine learning and logistic regression models in predicting acute kidney injury: A systematic review and meta-analysis. *Int. J. Med. Inform.* **2021**, *151*, 104484. [CrossRef]
21. Aminsharifi, A.; Irani, D.; Tayebi, S.; Jafari Kafash, T.; Shabanian, T.; Parsaei, H. Predicting the Postoperative Outcome of Percutaneous Nephrolithotomy with Machine Learning System: Software Validation and Comparative Analysis with Guy's Stone Score and the CROES Nomogram. *J. Endourol.* **2020**, *34*, 692–699. [CrossRef]
22. Blum, E.S.; Porras, A.R.; Biggs, E.; Tabrizi, P.R.; Sussman, R.D.; Sprague, B.M.; Shalaby-Rana, E.; Majd, M.; Pohl, H.G.; Linguraru, M.G. Early Detection of ureteropelvic junction obstruction using signal analysis and machine learning: A dynamic solution to a dynamic problem. *J. Urol.* **2018**, *199*, 847–852. [CrossRef]

23. Kocak, B.; Yardimci, A.H.; Bektas, C.T.; Turkcanoglu, M.H.; Erdim, C.; Yucetas, U.; Koca, S.B.; Kilickesmez, O. Textural differences between renal cell carcinoma subtypes: Machine learning-based quantitative computed tomography texture analysis with independent external validation. *Eur. J. Radiol.* **2018**, *107*, 149–157. [CrossRef]
24. Feng, Z.; Rong, P.; Cao, P.; Zhou, Q.; Zhu, W.; Yan, Z.; Liu, Q.; Wang, W. Machine learning-based quantitative texture analysis of CT images of small renal masses: Differentiation of angiomyolipoma without visible fat from renal cell carcinoma. *Eur. Radiol.* **2018**, *28*, 1625–1633. [CrossRef]
25. Hasnain, Z.; Mason, J.; Gill, K.; Miranda, G.; Gill, I.S.; Kuhn, P.; Newton, P.K. Machine learning models for predicting post-cystectomy recurrence and survival in bladder cancer patients. *PLoS ONE* **2019**, *14*, e0210976. [CrossRef] [PubMed]
26. Deng, K.; Li, H.; Guan, Y. Treatment Stratification of Patients with Metastatic Castration-Resistant Prostate Cancer by Machine Learning. *Iscience* **2020**, *23*, 100804. [CrossRef] [PubMed]
27. Giamarellos-Bourboulis, E.J.; Opal, S.M. The role of genetics and antibodies in sepsis. *Ann. Transl. Med.* **2016**, *4*, 328. [CrossRef] [PubMed]

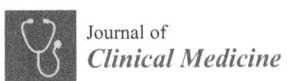

Article

Extracorporeal Shockwave Therapy (ESWT) Alleviates Pain, Enhances Erectile Function and Improves Quality of Life in Patients with Chronic Prostatitis/Chronic Pelvic Pain Syndrome

Wen-Ling Wu [1,2], Oluwaseun Adebayo Bamodu [1,3,4], Yuan-Hung Wang [4,5], Su-Wei Hu [1,2,5], Kai-Yi Tzou [1,2,6], Chi-Tai Yeh [4,7] and Chia-Chang Wu [1,2,6,*]

[1] Department of Urology, Shuang Ho Hospital, Taipei Medical University, New Taipei City 235, Taiwan; 15334@s.tmu.edu.tw (W.-L.W.); 16625@s.tmu.edu.tw (O.A.B.); 10352@s.tmu.edu.tw (S.-W.H.); 11579@s.tmu.edu.tw (K.-Y.T.)
[2] TMU Research Center of Urology and Kidney (TMU-RCUK), Taipei Medical University, Taipei City 110, Taiwan
[3] Department of Hematology and Oncology, Shuang Ho Hospital, Taipei Medical University, New Taipei City 235, Taiwan
[4] Department of Medical Research, Shuang Ho Hospital, Taipei Medical University, New Taipei City 235, Taiwan; d508091002@tmu.edu.tw (Y.-H.W.), ctyeh@s.tmu.edu.tw (C.-T.Y.)
[5] Graduate Institute of Clinical Medicine, College of Medicine, Taipei Medical University, Taipei 110, Taiwan
[6] Department of Urology, School of Medicine, College of Medicine, Taipei Medical University, Taipei City 110, Taiwan
[7] Department of Medical Laboratory Science and Biotechnology, Yuanpei University of Medical Technology, Hsinchu City 30015, Taiwan
* Correspondence: 08253@s.tmu.edu.tw; Tel.: +886-02-22490088 (ext. 8111); Fax: +886-02-2249-0088

Abstract: Purpose: Chronic prostatitis/chronic pelvic pain syndrome (CP/CPPS), affecting over 90% of patients with symptomatic prostatitis, remains a therapeutic challenge and adversely affects patients' quality of life (QoL). This study probed for likely beneficial effects of ESWT, evaluating its extent and durability. Patients and methods: Standardized indices, namely the pain, urinary, and QoL domains and total score of NIH-CPSI, IIEF-5, EHS, IPSS, and AUA QoL_US were employed in this study of patients with CP/CPPS who had been refractory to other prior treatments ($n = 215$; age range: 32–82 years; median age: 57.5 ± 12.4 years; modal age: 41 years). Results: For CP symptoms, the mean pre-ESWT NIH-CPSI total score of 27.1 ± 6.8 decreased by 31.3–53.6% over 12 months after ESWT. The mean pre-ESWT NIH-CPSI pain (12.5 ± 3.3), urinary (4.98 ± 2.7), and QoL (9.62 ± 2.1) domain scores improved by 2.3-fold, 2.2-fold, and 2.0-fold, respectively, by month 12 post-ESWT. Compared with the baseline IPSS of 13.9 ± 8.41, we recorded 27.1–50.9% amelioration of urinary symptoms during the 12 months post-ESWT. For erectile function, compared to pre-ESWT values, the IIEF-5 also improved by ~1.3-fold by month 12 after ESWT. This was corroborated by EHS of 3.11 ± 0.99, 3.37 ± 0.65, 3.42 ± 0.58, 3.75 ± 0.45, and 3.32 ± 0.85 at baseline, 1, 2, 6, and 12 months post-ESWT. Compared to the mean pre-ESWT QoL score (4.29 ± 1.54), the mean QoL values were 3.26 ± 1.93, 3.45 ± 2.34, 3.25 ± 1.69, and 2.6 ± 1.56 for months 1, 2, 6, and 12 after ESWT, respectively. Conclusions: This study shows ESWT, an outpatient and easy-to-perform, minimally invasive procedure, effectively alleviates pain, improves erectile function, and ameliorates quality of life in patients with refractory CP/CPPS.

Keywords: chronic prostatitis; chronic pelvic pain syndrome; extracorporeal shockwave therapy; ESWT; NIH-CPSI; EHS; IIEF-5; QoL

1. Introduction

Prostatitis affects an estimated 8.2% of the global population and remains a major health issue [1]. Added to the therapeutic challenge it poses to physicians, prostatitis adversely affect patients' quality of life (QoL) [2] and causes patients substantial economic constraint [3]. The National Institutes of Health (NIH) clinical syndromes-based classification system divides prostatitis into four categories: namely, category I, which includes acute systemic infection and replaces the so-called 'acute bacterial prostatitis'; category II, which replaces the erstwhile 'chronic bacterial prostatitis', and comprises recurrent urinary tract infection (UTI) in men with prostatic bacterial presence between infections; category III for chronic prostatitis/chronic pelvic pain syndrome (CP/CPPS), evidenced by chronic pelvic pain with no known alternative attributable pathology; and category IV for asymptomatic prostatitis based on biopsy- or semen analysis-confirmed inflammation [3–5].

Protracted painful prostatitis, herein termed CP/CPPS, affects over 90% of patients with symptomatic prostatitis [6], and is characterized by persistent or recurring pain/discomfort in the pelvis for at least 3 of the last 6 months, often accompanied by lower abdominal pain; painful ejaculation; genital pain; lower urinary tract symptoms (LUTS) such as hesitancy, straining, feeling of incomplete bladder emptying, poor or intermittent stream, dribbling, prolonged micturition, urgency, frequency, or nocturia; psycho-social impairments; and erectile/sexual dysfunction [3–6].

Over the last six decades, CP/CPPS, attributed to infection, inflammation, impaired urothelial integrity and function, endocrine imbalance, autoimmunity, voiding dysfunction, or neuropsychological factors [7,8], has remained a 'diagnosis of exclusion' with currently unclear or inexact underlying cause, thus stimulating interest and concerted research effort to demystify its etiology and unravel probable underlying molecular mechanisms. Recently, *Trichomonas Vaginalis* infection has been suggested as a probable pathoetiologic factor in CP/CPPS because of its complicity in chronic persistent prostatic infection and prostate epithelial cell inflammation [9]. Being able to cause inflammation by adhering to normal prostate epithelial cells [9,10], the association of *T. Vaginalis* with benign prostate hyperplasia (BPH) and prostate cancer is also currently being investigated [11,12]. However, the effect of *T. Vaginalis* on the development of chronic prostatitis remains unclear [13,14].

Despite advances in diagnostic and therapeutic approaches based on our evolving understanding of the CP/CPPS etiopathology, there is no international consensus-based approved single agent therapy with proven high efficacy against this syndrome [15], thus, the adoption of multi-modal approaches to treating CP/CPPS [16] such as the 'three As'. The 'three As' modality consists of α-blockers, antibiotics, and/or anti-inflammatory/immune modulation therapy. There is mounting evidence supporting the therapeutic efficacy of the three As in some patients with CP/CPPS [17]. The magnitude of effect and the disproportional mean decrease in the NIH Chronic Prostatitis Symptom Index (NIH—CPSI) and response rates in treatment groups in comparison to placebo groups suggest the superiority of directed multi-modal therapy over monotherapy, and advocate consideration of these agents for optimal management of patients with CP/CPPS [17]. Alternatively, phytotherapies, including quercetin, Cernilton, Eviprostat/pollen extract, and pentosane polysulfate [17,18], as well as non-pharmacological therapies such as acupuncture and extracorporeal shockwave therapy (ESWT), have also shown some efficacy in the treatment of CP/CPPS [8].

The UPOINTS algorithm, formed by addition of the sexuality (S) component to the original UPOINT system consisting of urinary domain (U), psycho-social (P), organ-specific (O), infection (I), neurological (*n*), and muscle tension and tenderness (T) domains, helps stratify patients into clusters of homogeneous clinical presentation, identifies recognizable phenotypes, and proposes specific treatment plans [19]. Accruing evidence indicates that treatment of patients consistent with this complex multi-modal disease phenotype-based therapeutic approach elicits clinically appreciable amelioration of CP/CPPS symptomatology in many patients, with the addition of second-line therapeutics such as 5-phosphodiesterase inhibitors, antidepressants, muscle relaxants, and anxiolytics to help elicit satisfactory treatment response in patients with sub-optimal response to initial first-line therapy [20]. There are reports associating the UPOINTS algorithm with clinical improvement in 75–84% of CP/CPPS cases [5,19–21].

As already mentioned, non-pharmacological therapies are also touted as effective against CP/CPPS [8,22]. ESWT is one such non-pharmacological treatment modality [22]. ESWT is well-known and widely used in urological clinics to treat Peyronie's disease, erectile dysfunction (ED), and chronic pelvic pain [23]. Zimmermann R. et al. first reported the use of ESWT for treating CP/CPPS in 2009. Their seminal report demonstrated the ease and safety of ESWT, as well as showed that all patients with CP/CPPS completed their treatment without complications and that follow-up was uneventful, with all treated patients exhibiting marked amelioration of pain, improved QoL, and better voiding conditions following ESWT, compared with progressive deterioration in the placebo group [24]. It has been suggested that the observed post-ESWT improvement in CP/CPPS may be due to "reducing passive muscle tone, hyperstimulating nociceptors, interrupting the flow of nerve impulses, or influencing the neuroplasticity of the pain memory" [25].

Despite these touted beneficial effects of ESWT on CP/CPPS, there are suggestions that its therapeutic effects may be short-lived, with tendency to decrease in month 6 of follow-up [23]. However, contradictory results on the effect of ESWT on CP/CPPS abound, especially with a dearth of long-term follow-up. Considering the short duration (3 months) of the premier ESWT study and the unusual lack of placebo response in the control group, as rightly posed by Marszalek M [25], outstanding questions linger regarding (i) suitable patient demographics or selection criteria for the treatment, (ii) the probable potentiating effect of previous treatment strategies, and (iii) the unclear durability of treatment benefit for lack of longer term effect data [23–25]. Thus, the present study evaluates the therapeutic effect of ESWT on CP/CPPS patients with prior treatment failure.

2. Methods

2.1. Patients

This single-center, prospective, single-arm cohort study was performed from September 2016 to January 2018 at the Shuang Ho Hospital, Taipei Medical University, New Taipei, Taiwan. A total of 215 patients with established diagnosis of CP/CPPS, non-inflammatory type (NIH type IIIb prostatitis), were included in our study. The study was approved by Taipei Medical University-Joint Institutional Review Board (Approval No.: N201712069), and written informed consent was obtained from all the enrolled patients. The study protocol was compliant with the Declaration of Helsinki.

Enrolled patients were seen in the outpatient settings. Diagnosis was established after thorough history-taking, physical examination, and screening with the following examinations: (i) urine analysis, (ii) urine culture, (iii) semen analysis, (iv) semen culture, (v) nucleic acid amplification test (NAAT) for *T. Vaginalis*, (vi) NAAT for *Chlamydia trichomatis*, (vii) blood test, including complete blood count/differential count, and C-reactive protein (CRP), (viii) prostate ultrasound, and (ix) kidney, ureter, and bladder (KUB) radiography.

2.2. Inclusion and Exclusion Criteria

Inclusion criteria were as follows: patients (i) aged 18 or above, (ii) diagnosed with CP/CPPS, (iii) suffered prostatitis-like symptoms for at least the last 6 months with no identifiable cause, (iv) refractory to administered medical therapies for at least the last 6 months. The exclusion criteria included (i) anatomical abnormalities of the genitourinary system, (ii) urinary tract or perineal region infection, (iii) cancer of the genitourinary system, (iv) prostate specific antigen >4, and (v) major surgery of the pelvic organs, including the prostate or rectum.

2.3. ESWT Protocol

All patients were treated in the dorsal recumbent position with perineal ESWT once a week for 6 consecutive weeks with a protocol of 3000 pulses at an energy of 0.25 mJoule/mm^2 and a frequency of 4 Hertz (Hz) using DUOLITH® SD1 (Storz Medical AG, Tägerwilen, Switzerland). Probe position was changed after every 500 pulses to broaden the therapy effect field, induce re-perfusion of the prostate, improve the hemodynamic profile of the prostatic artery, and forestall probable procedure-associated side-effects, such as, itchy or painful dysesthesia, ecchymosis, and petechiae. One cycle consisted of 6 sessions. The DUOLITH® SD1 is a mobile shockwave therapy apparatus with a SEPIA® hand-piece for ease of manipulation and positioning to facilitate focused shock waves.

2.4. Evaluation of Outcome

The primary outcomes of the present study, namely, pain reduction and amelioration of urinary symptoms, were evaluated using the NIH-CPSI, International Prostate Symptom Score (IPSS), and American Urological Association Quality of Life due to Urinary Symptoms (AUA QOL_US), while improved sexual function, being the secondary outcome, was assessed using the International Index of Erectile Function (IIEF), and Erection Hardness Score (EHS). All questionnaires were completed after detailed explanation during clinic visits (i) before commencing ESWT, (ii) after the third ESWT session, (iii) a week after the sixth ESWT session, (iv) 1 month, (v) 2 months, (vi) 6 months, and (vii) 12 months after the last ESWT session. Aside from ESWT treatment, all patients with concomitant *T. vaginalis* infection ($n = 19$) were given a single dose of 2 g Metronidazole. None of the enrolled subjects underwent transurethral resection of the prostate (TURP) during follow-up, nor did any receive other therapies concomitantly with ESWT.

2.5. Statistical Analyses

All statistical analyses were performed using IBM SPSS Statistics for Windows, Version 25.0 (IBM Corp. Released 2017, Armonk, NY, USA: IBM Corp). For randomly missing data, we used the pairwise deletion (also known as the 'available case analysis') by deleting any case with missing variables required for a specific analysis, but including such cases in analyses where all required variables were present. Pearson's chi-square (χ^2) test was used to determine the relationship or association between categorical variables. The paired sample t-test was used for comparing two dependent sample means, while the independent t-test was used to compare independent sample means. p values ≤ 0.05 were considered statistically significant.

3. Results

The present study evaluated the effect of ESWT on pain, erectile function, and QoL in patients with CP/CPPS ($n = 215$) using standardized evaluation indices, namely the pain domain, urinary domain, QoL domain, and total score of NIH-CPSI, IIEF-5, EHS, IPSS, and AUA QoL_US. Participants were aged 32–82 years (mean: 57.1 ± 12.41 years; median: 57.5 ± 12.41 years; modal age: 41 years).

For CP symptoms, the mean NIH-CPSI pain, urinary, and QoL domains, as well as total score before ESWT were 12.53 ± 3.25, 4.98 ± 2.72, 9.62 ± 2.06, and 27.10 ± 6.81, respectively. Compared to these baseline values, the mean NIH-CPSI total scores decreased by 31.3%, 37.3%, 35.7%, and 53.6% at 1, 2, 6, and 12 months after ESWT administration, respectively (Supplementary Table S1). Per component, we observed a 2.3-fold, 2.2-fold, and 2.0-fold improvement in the CPSI pain, urinary and QoL domains, respectively, by month 12 post-ESWT (Figure 1; also see Supplementary Table S1).

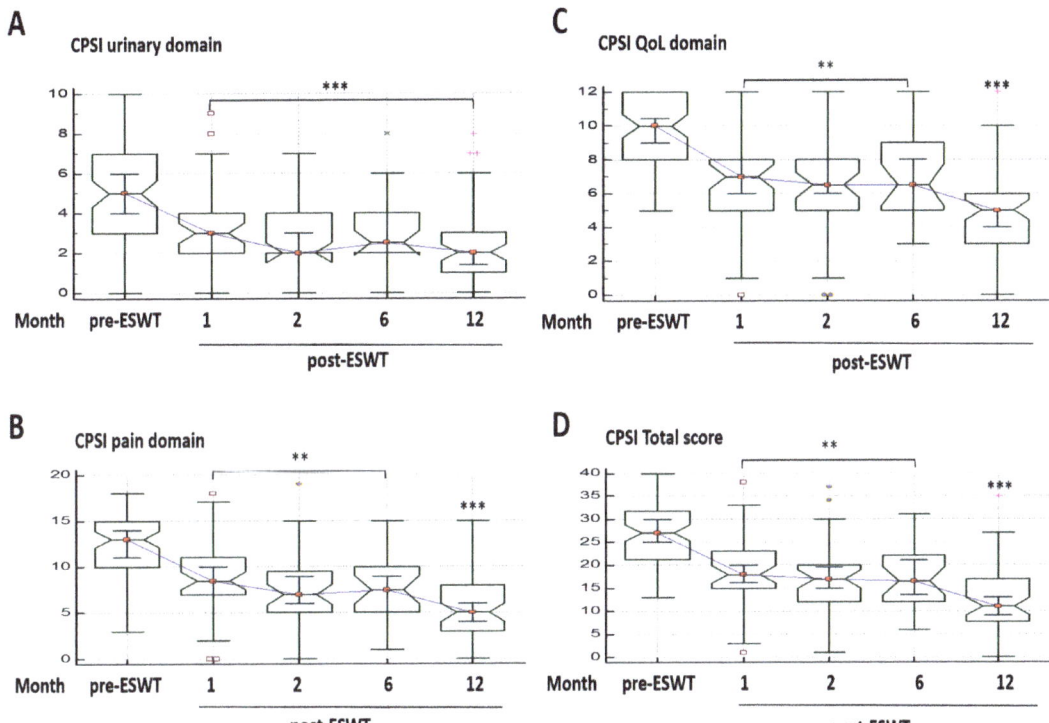

Figure 1. Extracorporeal Shockwave Therapy and Chronic Prostatitis Symptom Index (CPSI). Notched box-and-whiskers graphs showing the time-phased effect of extracorporeal shockwave therapy using the (**A**) urinary domain, (**B**) pain domain, (**C**) quality of life, and (**D**) total score over a period of 12 months. ** $p < 0.01$, *** $p < 0.001$.

For erectile function, the IIEF-5 also improved significantly after ESWT, as demonstrated by mean IIEF-5 scores of 18.43 ± 6.34 (1.1-fold), 20.42 ± 5.59 (1.3-fold), 20.25 ± 5.94 (1.3-fold), and 18.65 ± 6.85 (1.2-fold) at months 1, 2, 6, and 12 respectively, compared to the mean IIEF-5 score of 15.82 ± 7.70 before ESWT (Supplementary Table S1). This was corroborated by the improved EHS of 3.37 ± 0.65, 3.42 ± 0.58, 3.75 ± 0.45, and 3.32 ± 0.85 at 1, 2, 6, and 12 months post-ESWT, respectively, compared to baseline (3.11 ± 0.99) (Figure 2A,B; also see Supplementary Table S1).

Consistent with the NIH-CPSI, the severity of LUTS was ameliorated as measured by the IPSS. In comparison to the mean pre-ESWT IPSS of 13.9 ± 8.41, we recorded a 27.1%, 38.0%, 42.0%, and 50.9% time-dependent improvement, respectively, of urinary symptom severity at months 1, 2, 6, and 12 of ESWT (Figure 2C; Also see Supplementary Table S1).

Understanding that the severity of urinary symptoms, including pain, affects patients' QoL, we evaluated and demonstrated commensurate improvement in patients' QoL as per the AUA QOL_US. The mean QoL score before ESWT was 4.29 ± 1.54. For the first, second, sixth, and twelfth months following ESWT, we recorded mean QoL values of 3.26 ± 1.93, 3.45 ± 2.34, 3.25 ± 1.69, and 2.6 ± 1.56, respectively (Figure 2D; also see Table S1).

A baseline-normalized paired sample mean of all evaluated parameters is shown in Table 1. Compared to pre-ESWT status, ESWT elicited statistically significant improvement in all patients' clinical parameters ($p < 0.001$), except for the EHS at 2 months (mean baseline-paired difference = 0.23, $p = 0.096$), 6 months (mean baseline-paired difference = 0.25, $p = 0.351$), and 12 months (mean baseline-paired difference = 0.10, $p = 0.302$) following ESWT, compared to the 40.9% mean improvement in EHS ($p = 0.009$) at 1 month following ESWT (Table 1).

Table 1. Comparison of paired samples parameters over time.

Pair		n	Variable 1 (Mean ± SD)	Variable 2 (Mean ± SD)	Paired Differences			p-Value [a]
Variable 1	Variable 2				Mean ± SD	95% CI		
CPSI_urinary_domain_1	CPSI_urinary_domain_pESWT_1	41	4.32 ± 2.74	3.15 ± 2.17	−1.17 ± 1.87	−1.76 to −0.58		0.0003
CPSI_urinary_domain_1	CPSI_urinary_domain_pESWT_2	39	4.62 ± 2.75	2.82 ± 2.02	−1.79 ± 2.38	−2.56 to −1.03		<0.0001
CPSI_urinary_domain_1	CPSI_urinary_domain_pESWT_6	24	4.88 ± 2.63	2.88 ± 1.90	−2.00 ± 2.11	−2.90 to −1.11		0.0001
CPSI_urinary_domain_1	CPSI_urinary_domain_pESWT_12	59	4.85 ± 2.70	2.20 ± 1.92	−2.64 ± 2.66	−3.34 to −1.95		<0.0001
CPSI_pain_domain_1	CPSI_pain_domain_pESWT_1	41	11.85 ± 3.40	8.56 ± 4.30	−3.29 ± 3.72	−4.47 to −2.12		<0.0001
CPSI_pain_domain_1	CPSI_pain_domain_pESWT_2	39	12.36 ± 3.10	7.67 ± 4.23	−4.69 ± 4.40	−6.12 to −3.27		<0.0001
CPSI_pain_domain_1	CPSI_pain_domain_pESWT_6	24	12.29 ± 3.17	7.42 ± 3.86	−4.87 ± 4.01	−6.57 to −3.18		<0.0001
CPSI_pain_domain_1	CPSI_pain_domain_pESWT_12	59	12.29 ± 3.39	5.36 ± 3.62	−6.93 ± 4.45	−8.09 to −5.77		<0.0001
CPSI_QoL_domain_1	CPSI_QoL_domain_pESWT_1	41	9.27 ± 2.15	6.88 ± 2.87	−2.39 ± 2.96	−3.32 to −1.46		<0.0001
CPSI_QoL_domain_1	CPSI_QoL_domain_pESWT_2	39	9.51 ± 2.09	6.46 ± 2.96	−3.05 ± 3.15	−4.07 to −2.03		<0.0001
CPSI_QoL_domain_1	CPSI_QoL_domain_pESWT_6	24	9.42 ± 2.22	6.92 ± 2.80	−2.50 ± 2.47	−3.54 to −1.46		0.0001
CPSI_QoL_domain_1	CPSI_QoL_domain_pESWT_12	59	9.53 ± 2.05	4.85 ± 2.57	−4.68 ± 2.82	−5.41 to −3.94		<0.0001
CPSI_total_score_1	CPSI_total_score_pESWT_1	41	25.44 ± 6.96	18.59 ± 8.32	−6.85 ± 7.41	−9.19 to −4.52		<0.0001
CPSI_total_score_1	CPSI_total_score_pESWT_2	39	26.49 ± 6.77	16.95 ± 8.10	−9.54 ± 9.01	−12.46 to −6.62		<0.0001
CPSI_total_score_1	CPSI_total_score_pESWT_6	24	26.58 ± 7.03	17.21 ± 7.39	−9.38 ± 7.12	−12.38 to −6.37		<0.0001
CPSI_total_score_1	CPSI_total_score_pESWT_12	59	26.66 ± 6.95	12.37 ± 7.24	−14.29 ± 8.61	−16.53 to −12.04		<0.0001
EHS_1	EHS_pESWT_1	22	2.95 ± 1.17	3.36 ± 0.66	0.41 ± 0.67	0.11 to 0.70		0.009
EHS_1	EHS_pESWT_2	22	3.23 ± 0.97	3.45 ± 0.60	0.23 ± 0.61	−0.04 to 0.50		0.0961
EHS_1	EHS_pESWT_6	8	3.38 ± 0.74	3.63 ± 0.52	0.25 ± 0.71	−0.34 to 0.84		0.3506
EHS_1	EHS_pESWT_12	49	3.20 ± 0.82	3.31 ± 0.82	0.10 ± 0.68	−0.09 to 0.30		0.3019
IIEF_1	IIEF_pESWT_1	22	16.00 ± 7.89	18.36 ± 6.48	2.36 ± 3.13	0.98 to 3.75		0.0019
IIEF_1	IIEF_pESWT_2	22	18.14 ± 6.81	20.14 ± 5.77	2.00 ± 2.96	0.69 to 3.31		0.0046
IIEF_1	IIEF_pESWT_6	8	15.88 ± 7.86	19.50 ± 7.17	3.63 ± 3.93	0.34 to 6.91		0.0348
IIEF_1	IIEF_pESWT_12	50	17.06 ± 6.60	18.80 ± 6.53	1.74 ± 3.06	0.87 to 2.61		0.0002
IPSS_1	IPSS_pESWT_1	27	13.59 ± 8.31	10.37 ± 8.39	−3.22 ± 5.06	−5.23 to −1.22		0.0028
IPSS_1	IPSS_pESWT_2	27	13.81 ± 7.92	8.85 ± 5.95	−4.96 ± 5.99	−7.33 to −2.59		0.0002
IPSS_1	IPSS_pESWT_6	14	16.79 ± 9.21	7.93 ± 4.57	−8.86 ± 6.50	−12.61 to −5.10		0.0002
IPSS_1	IPSS_pESWT_12	56	13.71 ± 8.46	6.88 ± 5.14	−6.84 ± 6.29	−8.52 to −5.15		<0.0001
QoL_1	QoL_pESWT_1	26	4.04 ± 1.66	3.35 ± 1.92	−0.69 ± 1.69	−1.38 to −0.01		0.0473
QoL_1	QoL_pESWT_2	27	4.37 ± 1.42	3.48 ± 2.41	−0.89 ± 2.06	−1.71 to −0.07		0.0339
QoL_1	QoL_pESWT_6	14	5.14 ± 0.95	3.21 ± 1.72	−1.93 ± 1.33	−2.70 to −1.16		0.0001
QoL_1	QoL_pESWT_12	56	4.25 ± 1.59	2.61 ± 1.57	−1.64 ± 1.59	−2.07 to −1.22		<0.0001

[a]: Paired samples t-test; CPSI/NIH-CPSI = National Institute of Health Chronic Prostatitis Symptom Index; 95% CI = 95% confidence interval; SD = standard deviation; VAS = visual analog scale; IPSS = International Prostate Symptom Score; QoL/AUA QoL_US = American Urological Association Quality of Life Due to Urinary Symptoms; IIEF = International Index of Erectile Function; EHS = erectile hardness score; ESWT = extracorporeal shockwave therapy; pESWT = post-extracorporeal shockwave therapy.

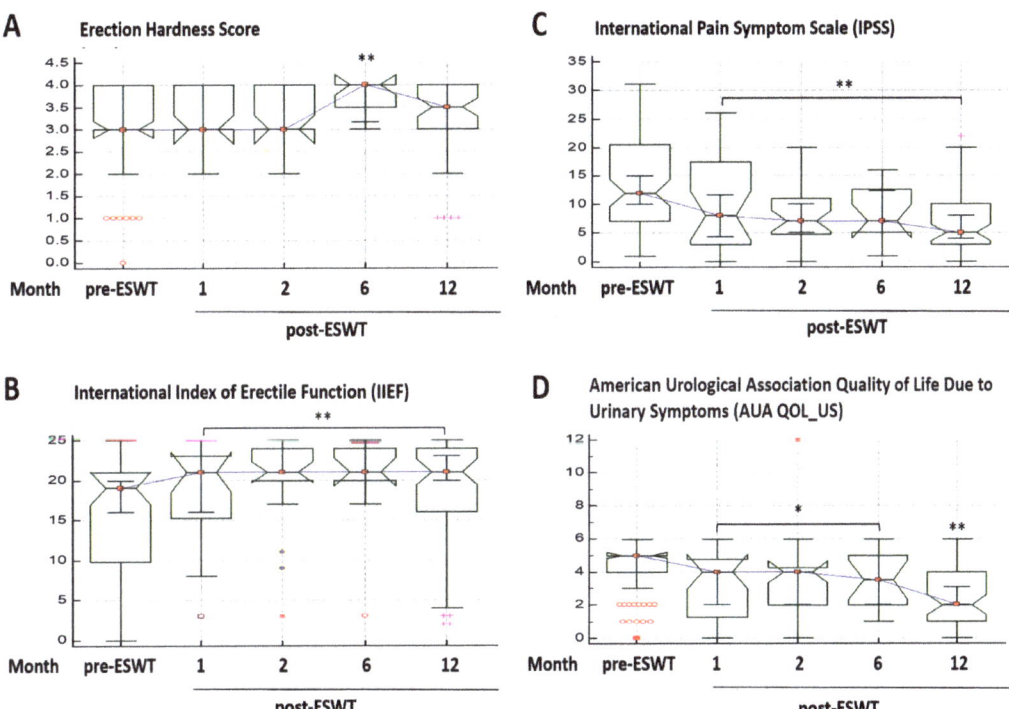

Figure 2. Effect of extracorporeal shockwave therapy in patients with chronic prostatitis/chronic pelvic pain syndrome (CP/CPSS). Notched box-and-whiskers graphs showing the time-phased effect of extracorporeal shockwave therapy on the (**A**) erection hardness score, (**B**) international index of erectile function, (**C**) international pain symptom scale, and (**D**) American Urological Association Quality of Life due to Urinary Symptoms over a period of 12 months. * $p < 0.05$, ** $p < 0.01$.

4. Discussion

In the past decades, several studies across different medical disciplines have indicated the therapeutic efficacy of ESWT to various degrees against diverse medial conditions, including spasticity after upper motor neuron injury [26], tendinopathies, musculoskeletal conditions and soft tissue disorders [27–32], refractory angina pectoris [33], erectile dysfunction [34], and sexual conditions other than erectile dysfunction [35,36]. While several studies have also suggested that the use of ESWT exerts a beneficial effect in patients with CP/CPPS [8,15–24], as with erectile dysfunction [37], the application of ESWT in the management of CP/CPPS is not without its controversies [23,25].

Although ESWT has been touted as a major therapeutic advance in the field of CP/CPPS in recent decades, as briefly summarized in Table 2, it remains far from being a perfect treatment paradigm and harbors certain limitations as already alluded to earlier [23–25].

Table 2. Review of previous studies on ESWT in patients with CP/CPPS.

Study	Study Design	No. of Patients	Baseline NIH-CPSI Score	Intervention: ESWT	Treatment Duration	Follow-Up (Weeks)	Outcome (at the End of Follow-Up)
Rayegani 2020	RCT	31	27.87 ± 7.2	4 sessions of focused ESWT (a protocol of 3000 impulses, 0.25 mJ/mm² and 3 Hz of frequency)	Once a week for 4 weeks	1, 4, 12	NIH-CPSI (↓), VAS (↓), Qmax (↑), PVR (↓), IPSS (↓), IIEF (↓), NIH QOL (↑)
Zhang 2019	Non-RCT	45	28.52 ± 4.07	rESWT (3000 pulses each; pressure: 1.8–2.0 bar; frequency: 10 Hz)	Once a week for 8 weeks	1, 4, 8, 12	NIH-CPSI (↓), VAS (↓), IPSS (↓), IIEF (↑), NIH QOL (↓)
Guu 2018	Cohort	33	28.03 ± 6.18	3000 impulses at a frequency of 4 Hz, with a energy density of 0.25 mJ/mm²	Once a week for 4 weeks	1, 4, 12	NIH-CPSI (↓), VAS (↓), IPSS (↓), IIEF-5 (↑), EHS(–), IELT(–)
Salecha 2017	Cohort	50	NA	2500 impulses	Once a week for 4 weeks	1, 4, 12	NIH-CPSI, VAS (↓), ultrasound, PSA level
Letizia 2017	Cohort	39	NA	NA	Once a week for 6 weeks	1, 6, 12	pain score, urinary score, quality-of-life (NIH-CPSI?)
Al Edwan 2017 (1 year follow up of Mohammad 2016?)	Cohort	41	27.7 ± 7.6	2500 impulses at a frequency of 3 Hz, with a energy density of 0.25 mJ/mm²	Once a week for 4 weeks	2, 6 months, 12 months	NIH-CPSI (↓), IPSS (↓), AUA QOL_US (↓), IIEF (↑)
Turcan 2016	Cohort	20	NA	Frequency of 8 Hz	4 times weekly for ?	4, 26	NIH-CPSI
Pajovic 2016	RCT	30	31.06 ± 7.75	3000 impulses at a frequency of 3 Hz, with a energy density of 0.25 mJ/mm²	Once a week for 4 weeks	12, 24	NIH-CPSI (↓), ultrasound
Mohammad 2016	Cohort	25	NA	2500 impulses over 13 min	Once a week for 4 weeks	2	NIH-CPSI (↓), IPSS (↓), AUA QOL_US (↓), IIEF (↑)
Kulchavenya 2016	Cohort	27	NA	2000–3000 impulses with a energy density of 0.056–0.085 mJ/mm²	Twice weekly for 3 weeks	1, 4	NIH-CPSI (↓), LDF
Moayednia 2014	RCT	19	26.03 ± 3.72	3000 impulses at a frequency of 3 Hz, with a energy density of 0.25 mJ/mm²	Once a week for 4 weeks	16, 20, 24	NIH-CPSI(–), VAS(–)

Table 2. Cont.

Study	Study Design	No. of Patients	Baseline NIH-CPSI Score	Intervention: ESWT	Treatment Duration	Follow-Up (Weeks)	Outcome (at the End of Follow-Up)
Vahdatpour 2013	RCT	40	26.5 ± 3.4	3000 impulses at a frequency of 3 Hz, with a energy density of 0.25–0.4 mJ/mm^2	Once a week for 4 weeks	1, 2, 3, 12	NIH-CPSI(−), VAS(?)
Kernesiuk 2013	Cohort	15	NA	NA	Once a week for 4 weeks	1, 2, 4, 12	NIH-CPSI(↓)in QOL and pain domain)
Zeng 2012	RCT	40	30.5 ± 4.7	2000 impulses at a frequency of 2 Hz, with a energy density of 0.06 mJ/mm^2- max tolerated dose	5 times weekly for 2 weeks	4, 12	NIH-CPSI (↓)
Mathers 2011	Cohort	14	26.1 ± 1.8	NA	Once a week for at least 3 weeks	4, 12	NIH-CPSI (↓)
Zimmermann 2010 (1 year follow up Zimmermann 2009)	RCT	44	NA	3000 impulses at a frequency of 3 Hz, with a energy density of 0.25 mJ/mm^2		1, 3, 6, 12 months	NIH-CPSI, VAS, IPSS, IIEF
Zimmermann 2009	RCT	30	23.20 ± 0.66	3000 impulses at a frequency of 3 Hz, with a energy density of 0.25 mJ/mm^2	Once a week for 4 weeks	1, 4, 12	NIH-CPSI (↓), VAS (↓), IPSS (↓), IIEF (↑)
Zimmermann 2008	Cohort Study	14	10.0	2000 impulses at a frequency of 3 Hz, with a energy density of 0.11 mJ/mm^2	3 times weekly for 2 weeks	1, 4, 12	NIH-CPSI, VAS, IPS
		20	19.9	3000 impulses at a frequency of 3 Hz, with a energy density of 0.25 mJ/mm^2	Once a week for 4 weeks	1, 4, 12	SNIH-CPSI (↓), VAS (↓), IPSS(−)

ESWT: extracorporeal shock wave therapy, rESWT: radial extracorporeal shock wave therapy; CP/CPPS: chronic pain/chronic pelvic pain syndrome, NIH-CPSI: national institute of health-chronic prostatitis symptom index, VAS: visual analogue scale, IIEF-5: 5-item version of the international index of erectie function, EHS: erection hardness score, IELT: intravaginal ejaculation latency time, AUA QOL_US: American urological association quality of life due to urinary symptoms, Qmax: maximum flow rate; PVR: post-void residual urine; LDF: laser Doppler flowmetry, (↓): statistical significance decrease ($p < 0.05$), (↑): statistical significance increase ($p < 0.05$), (−): no statistical difference ($p > 0.05$), NA: not available. Question mark (?) implies lack of certainty, as the cited study itself lacked clarity on the association.

The present study demonstrated the beneficial effect of ESWT on pain, erectile function, and QoL in patients with CP/CPPS ($n = 215$) at our facility based on improved pain domain, urinary domain, QoL domain, and total score of NIH-CPSI, IIEF-5, EHS, IPSS, and AUA QoL_US. Our findings are consistent with those of Yuan P. et al.'s meta-analysis, which demonstrated that low-intensity ESWT (Li-ESWT) was significantly efficacious in treating patients with CP/CPPS throughout the follow-up of 4 and 12 weeks, as well as at the 24-week endpoint, despite the statistically insignificant effect difference at 24-week follow-up due to insufficient data [38].

In our study, we demonstrated significant alleviation of pain in patients after ESWT. As mentioned by Zimmerman R et al. [24], the observed pain alleviation may be attributed to intracellular alterations following conversion of the mechanical extracorporeal shock-waves to biochemical signals. In addition to enhanced local microvascularization, coupled with reduced residual muscle tension and spasticity [24], we posit that the pulsatile stimulation of pain receptors (nociceptors) by ESWT disrupts in part or completely impedes the transmission of potential pain stimuli; it is also probable that ESWT simply overstimulates the nociceptors beyond their sensitivity threshold with consequent numbing of the sensory neurons to noxious stimuli, thus resulting in reduced pain perception. Concordant with the "neural pain memory" hypothesis put forward by Wess OJ [39], it is also conceivable that due to the plasticity of synapses, ESWT possibly effaces the noxious link established between pain sensory input and motor nerve signal output, and thereby reverses the sensation of chronic pain. Essentially, ESWT elicits the alleviation of pain by selectively eliminating pathological reflex patterns [24,39].

Furthermore, apart from pain alleviation, we also demonstrated that ESWT ameliorated the severity of other prostatitis symptoms in our CP/CPPS cohort with a 53.6% decrease in NIH-CPSI, 17.9% increase in IIEF-5, 6.8% increase in EHS, and 50.9% decrease in IPSS by month 12 after ESWT, concordant with the beneficial effect of ESWT in patients with CPPS (17% decrease in NIH-CPSI, 5.3% increase in IIEF, and 25% decrease in IPSS) reported by Zimmerman R et al. by month 3 after ESWT [24]. Additionally, this is consistent with the conclusions of a recent meta-analysis that "-ESWT showed great efficacy for the treatment of CP/CPPS at the endpoint and during the follow-up of 4 and 12 weeks" [38].

Moreover, because CP/CPPS-pathognomonic ED and LUTS significantly affect QoL, we demonstrated that ESWT improves the QoL of patients with CP/CPPS. This aligns with Zimmermann R et al.'s findings [24], and with reports that over 80% of patients that were non-responsive to therapy responded to ESWT by month 3, thus projecting ESWT as a salvage or rescue treatment for restoring clinical ability and improving QoL in patients with CP/CPPS who were refractory to the traditional 'three As' therapy [40]. In addition, Yan X, et al. [41] also documented significant improvement in all domains of the NIH-CPSI, including the QoL domain, and in the QoL as per the AUA QoL_US.

A major strength of this study is that unlike most studies on the effect of ESWT on CP/CPPS, where the mean follow-up duration was 12 weeks (month 3) after ESWT, the present study followed patients up to 48 weeks (month 12) post-ESWT in order to rule out suggestions that the post-ESWT beneficial effects were transient or short-term. To the best of our knowledge, this is the longest documented follow-up duration for any study on the effect of ESWT in patients with CP/CPPS. Nevertheless, more studies exploring the long-term durability of ESWT efficacy and the safety profile across all standard clinical indices are warranted. Having said that, aside from one case of post-procedure dysesthesia, which was transient and mild, our results and observations indicate that ESWT is a safe treatment for CP/CPPS, as follow-up was uneventful, with no aggravated complications recorded through the entire 48 weeks of follow-up. None of the participants opted out of the study due to any reported treatment-related complication. Consistent with contemporary knowledge and documented reports, long-term complications of ESWT are unknown.

Like many studies of this nature, the present study has some limitations, including being a single-center study, thus prone to being critiqued for lack of external validation or the scientific rigor necessary for widespread generalization or consensus. Secondly, this was a prospective, single-arm cohort study, thus lacking a control or sham group for comparison and exclusion of placebo effect. Thirdly, the cohort size of 215 patients with CP/CPPS, though greater than the minimum necessary number (i.e., given an expected average improvement in CPSI total score of 5 points, the sample size required was 14 ($\alpha = 0.05$, $\beta = 0.8$, $\sigma = 6$)) to meet the required statistical constraints, was relatively small and carried the risk of not representing CP/CPPS of all known pathoetiologies, thus necessitating the evaluation of the efficacy of ESWT in larger and multi-center cohort studies.

5. Conclusions

As summarized in our schematic abstract (Figure 3), the present study demonstrated that ESWT, an outpatient and easy-to-perform, minimally invasive procedure, effectively alleviates pain, improves erectile function, and ameliorates quality of life in patients with CP/CPPS. Our study highlighted the putative ability of ESWT to reverse the pathophysiology of CP/CPPS at the cellular level, elicit durable improvement in patients' clinical status, and restore spontaneous erectile function, with minimal or null side effects.

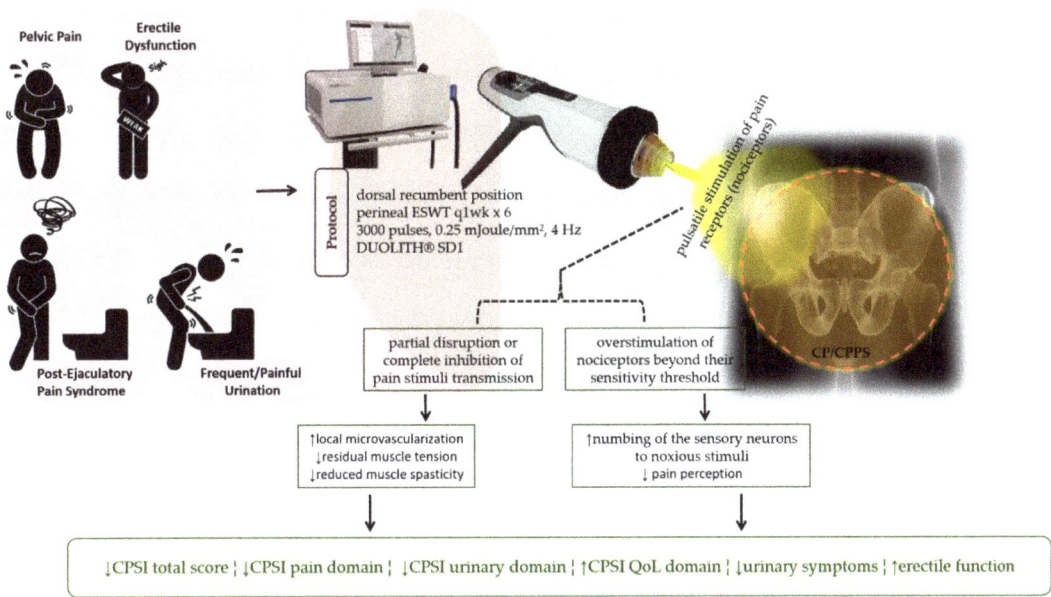

Figure 3. Schematic abstract: By disrupting pain stimuli transmission or overstimulation of nociceptors, ESWT effectively alleviates pain, improves erectile function, and ameliorates quality of life in patients with CP/CPPS through increased re-perfusion and numbing of sensory neurons to noxious stimuli, with associated reduction in residual muscle tension, spasticity, and pain perception.

Supplementary Materials: The following are available online at https://www.mdpi.com/article/10.3390/jcm10163602/s1, Table S1: Baseline and time-phased changes in NIH-CPSI, IIEF-5, EHS, IPSS and AUA QOL_US Scores in participants ($n = 215$).

Author Contributions: W.-L.W., O.A.B., C.-C.W.—Study conception and design, collection and assembly of data, data analysis and interpretation, and manuscript writing. Y.-H.W., S.-W.H., K.-Y.T., C.-T.Y.—Data analysis and interpretation. O.A.B., Y.-H.W., C.-C.W.—Provision of resources and administrative oversight. All authors have read and agreed to the published version of the manuscript.

Funding: This study received no external funding.

Institutional Review Board Statement: The study was approved by Taipei Medical University-Joint Institutional Review Board (Approval no.: N201712069), and written informed consent was obtained from all the enrolled patients. The study protocol was compliant with the Declaration of Helsinki.

Informed Consent Statement: Informed consent was obtained from all subjects involved in the study.

Data Availability Statement: The data used and analyzed in the current study are available on request from the corresponding author.

Acknowledgments: The authors thank all attending physicians from the Department of Urology, Shuang Ho Hospital, Taipei Medical University, for their assistance with patients' data collation.

Conflicts of Interest: The authors declare that they have no conflict of interest.

Abbreviations

AUA	American Urological Association
CP/CPPS	Chronic prostatitis/chronic pelvic pain syndrome
CPSI	Chronic Prostatitis Symptom Index
ED	Erectile dysfunction
EHS	Erection hardness score
ESWT	Extracorporeal shockwave therapy
IIEF-5	International Index of Erectile Function (simplified)
IPSS	International Prostate Symptom Score
LUTS	Lower urinary tract symptoms
NIH	National Institutes of Health
QoL	Quality of life

References

1. Krieger, J.N.; Lee, S.W.H.; Jeon, J.; Cheah, P.Y.; Liong, M.L.; Riley, D.E. Epidemiology of prostatitis. *Int. J. Antimicrob. Agents* **2008**, *31* (Suppl. 1), S85–S90. [CrossRef]
2. Collins, M.M.; Pontari, M.A.; O'Leary, M.P.; Calhoun, E.A.; Santanna, J.; Landis, J.R.; Kusek, J.W.; Litwin, M. Quality of life is impaired in men with chronic prostatitis: The Chronic Prostatitis Collaborative Research Network. *J. Gen. Intern. Med.* **2001**, *16*, 656–662. [CrossRef]
3. Lepor, H. Pathophysiology of Lower Urinary Tract Symptoms in the Aging Male Population. *Rev. Urol.* **2005**, *7*, S3–S11.
4. Magistro, G.; Stief, C.G.; Wagenlehner, F.M.E. Chronische Prostatitis/chronisches Beckenschmerzsyndrom. *Der Urol.* **2020**, *59*, 739–748. [CrossRef] [PubMed]
5. Polackwich, A.S.; Shoskes, D.A. Chronic prostatitis/chronic pelvic pain syndrome: A review of evaluation and therapy. *Prostate Cancer Prostatic Dis.* **2016**, *19*, 132–138. [CrossRef]
6. Krieger, J.N. NIH Consensus Definition and Classification of Prostatitis. *JAMA* **1999**, *282*, 236–237. [CrossRef]
7. Breser, M.L.; Salazar, F.C.; Rivero, V.E.; Motrich, R.D. Immunological Mechanisms Underlying Chronic Pelvic Pain and Prostate Inflammation in Chronic Pelvic Pain Syndrome. *Front. Immunol.* **2017**, *8*, 898. [CrossRef] [PubMed]
8. Franco, J.V.; Turk, T.; Jung, J.H.; Xiao, Y.-T.; Iakhno, S.; Garrote, V.; Vietto, V. Non-pharmacological interventions for treating chronic prostatitis/chronic pelvic pain syndrome. *Cochrane Database Syst. Rev.* **2018**, *2018*, CD012551. [CrossRef]
9. Kim, J.-H.; Han, I.-H.; Kim, S.-S.; Park, S.-J.; Min, D.-Y.; Ahn, M.-H.; Ryu, J.-S. Interaction between Trichomonas vaginalis and the Prostate Epithelium. *Korean J. Parasitol.* **2017**, *55*, 213–218. [CrossRef]
10. Iqbal, J.; Al-Rashed, J.; Kehinde, E.O. Detection of Trichomonas vaginalis in prostate tissue and serostasin in patients with asymptomatic benign prostatic hyperplasia. *BMC Infect. Dis.* **2016**, *16*, 506. [CrossRef] [PubMed]
11. Zhu, Z.; Davidson, K.T.; Brittingham, A.; Wakefield, M.; Bai, Q.; Xiao, H.; Fang, Y. Trichomonas vaginalis: A possible foe to prostate cancer. *Med. Oncol.* **2016**, *33*, 115. [CrossRef] [PubMed]
12. Han, I.; Kim, J.; Jang, K.; Ryu, J. Inflammatory mediators of prostate epithelial cells stimulated with Trichomonas vaginalis promote proliferative and invasive properties of prostate cancer cells. *Prostate* **2019**, *79*, 1133–1146. [CrossRef]
13. Papeš, D.; Pasini, M.; Jeroncic, A.; Vargović, M.; Kotarski, V.; Markotić, A.; Škerk, V. Detection of sexually transmitted pathogens in patients with chronic prostatitis/chronic pelvic pain: A prospective clinical study. *Int. J. STD AIDS* **2017**, *28*, 613–615. [CrossRef] [PubMed]
14. Im, S.; Han, I.; Kim, J.; Gu, N.; Seo, M.; Chung, Y.; Ryu, J. Inflammatory response of a prostate stromal cell line induced by Trichomonas vaginalis. *Parasite Immunol.* **2016**, *38*, 218–227. [CrossRef]

15. Nickel, J.C.; Shoskes, D.A.; Wagenlehner, F.M.E. Management of chronic prostatitis/chronic pelvic pain syndrome (CP/CPPS): The studies, the evidence, and the impact. *World J. Urol.* **2013**, *31*, 747–753. [CrossRef]
16. Magistro, G.; Wagenlehner, F.M.; Grabe, M.; Weidner, W.; Stief, C.G.; Nickel, J.C. Contemporary Management of Chronic Prostatitis/Chronic Pelvic Pain Syndrome. *Eur. Urol.* **2016**, *69*, 286–297. [CrossRef]
17. Thakkinstian, A.; Attia, J.; Anothaisintawee, T.; Nickel, J.C. α-blockers, antibiotics and anti-inflammatories have a role in the management of chronic prostatitis/chronic pelvic pain syndrome. *BJU Int.* **2012**, *110*, 1014–1022. [CrossRef]
18. Sandhu, J.; Tu, H.Y.V. Recent advances in managing chronic prostatitis/chronic pelvic pain syndrome. *F1000Research* **2017**, *6*, 1747. [CrossRef]
19. Magri, V.; Boltri, M.; Cai, T.; Colombo, R.; Cuzzocrea, S.; De Visschere, P.; Giuberti, R.; Granatieri, C.M.; Latino, M.A.; Larganà, G.; et al. Multidisciplinary approach to prostatitis. *Arch. Ital. Urol. Androl.* **2018**, *90*, 227–248. [CrossRef] [PubMed]
20. Magri, V.; Marras, E.; Restelli, A.; Wagenlehner, F.M.; Perletti, G. Multimodal therapy for category III chronic prostatitis/chronic pelvic pain syndrome in UPOINTS phenotyped patients. *Exp. Ther. Med.* **2015**, *9*, 658–666. [CrossRef]
21. Shoskes, D.A.; Nickel, J.C.; Kattan, M. Phenotypically Directed Multimodal Therapy for Chronic Prostatitis/Chronic Pelvic Pain Syndrome: A Prospective Study Using UPOINT. *Urology* **2010**, *75*, 1249–1253. [CrossRef] [PubMed]
22. Franco, J.V.A.; Turk, T.; Jung, J.H.; Xiao, Y.-T.; Iakhno, S.; Garrote, V.; Vietto, V. Non-pharmacological interventions for treating chronic prostatitis/chronic pelvic pain syndrome: A Cochrane systematic review. *BJU Int.* **2019**, *124*, 197–208. [CrossRef]
23. Fojecki, G.L.; Tiessen, S.; Osther, P.J.S. Extracorporeal shock wave therapy (ESWT) in urology: A systematic review of outcome in Peyronie's disease, erectile dysfunction and chronic pelvic pain. *World J. Urol.* **2016**, *35*, 1–9. [CrossRef] [PubMed]
24. Zimmermann, R.; Cumpanas, A.; Miclea, F.; Janetschek, G. Extracorporeal Shock Wave Therapy for the Treatment of Chronic Pelvic Pain Syndrome in Males: A Randomised, Double-Blind, Placebo-Controlled Study. *Eur. Urol.* **2009**, *56*, 418–424. [CrossRef]
25. Marszalek, M.; Berger, I.; Madersbacher, S. Low-Energy Extracorporeal Shock Wave Therapy for Chronic Pelvic Pain Syndrome: Finally, the Magic Bullet? *Eur. Urol.* **2009**, *56*, 425–426. [CrossRef]
26. Liu, D.-Y.; Zhong, D.; Li, J.; Jin, R.-J. The effectiveness and safety of extracorporeal shock wave therapy (ESWT) on spasticity after upper motor neuron injury. *Medicine* **2020**, *99*, e18932. [CrossRef]
27. Stania, M.; Juras, G.; Chmielewska, D.; Polak, A.; Kucio, C.; Król, P. Extracorporeal Shock Wave Therapy for Achilles Tendinopathy. *BioMed Res. Int.* **2019**, *2019*, 1–13. [CrossRef] [PubMed]
28. Vitali, M.; Rodriguez, N.N.; Pironti, P.; Drossinos, A.; Di Carlo, G.; Chawla, A.; Gianfranco, F. ESWT and nutraceutical supplementation (Tendisulfur Forte) vs ESWT-only in the treatment of lateral epicondylitis, Achilles tendinopathy, and rotator cuff tendinopathy: A comparative study. *J. Drug Assess.* **2019**, *8*, 77–86. [CrossRef]
29. Mishra, B.N.; Poudel, R.R.; Banskota, B.; Shrestha, B.K.; Banskota, A.K. Effectiveness of extra-corporeal shock wave therapy (ESWT) vs methylprednisolone injections in plantar fasciitis. *J. Clin. Orthop. Trauma* **2019**, *10*, 401–405. [CrossRef]
30. Yan, C.; Xiong, Y.; Chen, L.; Endo, Y.; Hu, L.; Liu, M.; Liu, J.; Xue, H.; Abududilibaier, A.; Mi, B.; et al. A comparative study of the efficacy of ultrasonics and extracorporeal shock wave in the treatment of tennis elbow: A meta-analysis of randomized controlled trials. *J. Orthop. Surg. Res.* **2019**, *14*, 248. [CrossRef]
31. Liao, C.-D.; Xie, G.-M.; Tsauo, J.-Y.; Chen, H.-C.; Liou, T.-H. Efficacy of extracorporeal shock wave therapy for knee tendinopathies and other soft tissue disorders: A meta-analysis of randomized controlled trials. *BMC Musculoskelet. Disord.* **2018**, *19*, 278. [CrossRef]
32. Reilly, J.M.; Bluman, E.; Tenforde, A.S. Effect of Shockwave Treatment for Management of Upper and Lower Extremity Musculoskeletal Conditions: A Narrative Review. *PM&R* **2018**, *10*, 1385–1403. [CrossRef]
33. Slavich, M.; Pizzetti, G.; Vella, A.M.; Carlucci, C.; Margonato, D.; Spoladore, R.; Fragasso, G.; Margonato, A. Extracorporeal myocardial shockwave therapy; a precious blast for refractory angina patients. *Cardiovasc. Revasc. Med.* **2018**, *19*, 263–267. [CrossRef]
34. Usta, M.F.; Gabrielson, A.T.; Bivalacqua, T.J. Low-intensity extracorporeal shockwave therapy in the treatment of erectile dysfunction following radical prostatectomy: A critical review. *Int. J. Impot. Res.* **2019**, *31*, 231–238. [CrossRef]
35. Fode, M.; Russo, G.I.; Verze, P. Therapeutic areas of Li-ESWT in sexual medicine other than erectile dysfunction. *Int. J. Impot. Res.* **2019**, *31*, 223–230. [CrossRef] [PubMed]
36. Porst, H. Review of the Current Status of Low Intensity Extracorporeal Shockwave Therapy (Li-ESWT) in Erectile Dysfunction (ED), Peyronie's Disease (PD), and Sexual Rehabilitation After Radical Prostatectomy with Special Focus on Technical Aspects of the Different Marketed ESWT Devices Including Personal Experiences in 350 Patients. *Sex. Med. Rev.* **2021**, *9*, 93–122. [CrossRef]
37. Yang, H.; Seftel, A.D. Controversies in low intensity extracorporeal shockwave therapy for erectile dysfunction. *Int. J. Impot. Res.* **2019**, *31*, 239–242. [CrossRef]
38. Yuan, P.; Ma, D.; Zhang, Y.; Gao, X.; Liu, Z.; Li, R.; Wang, T.; Wang, S.; Liu, J.; Liu, X. Efficacy of low-intensity extracorporeal shock wave therapy for the treatment of chronic prostatitis/chronic pelvic pain syndrome: A systematic review and meta-analysis. *Neurourol. Urodyn.* **2019**, *38*, 1457–1466. [CrossRef] [PubMed]
39. Wess, O.J. Chronic pain and pain relief by extracorporeal shock wave therapy. *Urol. Res.* **2011**, *39*, 515–519. [CrossRef] [PubMed]
40. Guu, S.-J.; Geng, J.-H.; Chao, I.-T.; Lin, H.-T.; Lee, Y.-C.; Juan, Y.-S.; Liu, C.-C.; Wang, C.-J.; Tsai, C.-C. Efficacy of Low-Intensity Extracorporeal Shock Wave Therapy on Men with Chronic Pelvic Pain Syndrome Refractory to 3-As Therapy. *Am. J. Men's Health* **2017**, *12*, 441–452. [CrossRef] [PubMed]
41. Yan, X.; Yang, G.; Cheng, L.; Chen, M.; Cheng, X.; Chai, Y.; Luo, C.; Zeng, B. [Effect of extracorporeal shock wave therapy on diabetic chronic wound healing and its histological features]. *Zhongguo Xiu Fu Chong Jian Wai Ke Za Zhi* **2012**, *26*, 961–967. [PubMed]

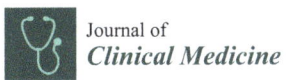

Article

Comparison of Holmium:YAG and Thulium Fiber Lasers on the Risk of Laser Fiber Fracture

Audrey Uzan [1,2], Paul Chiron [1,2], Frédéric Panthier [1,2], Mattieu Haddad [1,2], Laurent Berthe [3], Olivier Traxer [1,2] and Steeve Doizi [1,2,*]

[1] Sorbonne Université, GRC n°20, Groupe de Recherche Clinique sur la Lithiase Urinaire, Hôpital Tenon, F-75020 Paris, France; audrey.uzan@aphp.fr (A.U.); p.chiron@laposte.net (P.C.); frederic.panthier@aphp.fr (F.P.); mattieu.haddad@gmail.com (M.H.); olivier.traxer@aphp.fr (O.T.)
[2] Sorbonne Université, Service d'Urologie, AP-HP, Hôpital Tenon, F-75020 Paris, France
[3] PIMM, UMR 8006 CNRS-Arts et Métiers ParisTech, 151 bd de l'Hôpital, F-75013 Paris, France; laurent.berthe@ensam.eu
* Correspondence: steeve.doizi@aphp.fr; Tel.: +33-1-56-01-61-53; Fax: +33-1-56-01-63-77

Abstract: Objectives: To compare the risk of laser fiber fracture between Ho:YAG laser and Thulium Fiber Laser (TFL) with different laser fiber diameters, laser settings, and fiber bending radii. METHODS: Lengths of 200, 272, and 365 μm single use fibers were used with a 30 W Ho:YAG laser and a 50 W Super Pulsed TFL. Laser fibers of 150 μm length were also tested with the TFL only. Five different increasingly smaller bend radii were tested: 1, 0.9, 0.75, 0.6, and 0.45 cm. A total of 13 different laser settings were tested for the Ho:YAG laser: six fragmentation settings with a short pulse duration, and seven dusting settings with a long pulse duration. A total of 33 different laser settings were tested for the TFL. Three laser settings were common two both lasers: 0.5 J × 12 Hz, 0.8 J × 8 Hz, 2 J × 3 Hz. The laser was activated for 5 min or until fiber fracture. Each measurement was performed ten times. Results: While fiber failures occurred with all fiber diameters with Ho:YAG laser, none were reported with TFL. Identified risk factors of fiber fracture with the Ho:YAG laser were short pulse and high energy for the 365 μm fibers ($p = 0.041$), but not for the 200 and 272 μm fibers ($p = 1$ and $p = 0.43$, respectively). High frequency was not a risk factor of fiber fracture. Fiber diameter also seemed to be a risk factor of fracture. The 200 μm fibers broke more frequently than the 272 and 365 μm ones ($p = 0.039$). There was a trend for a higher number of fractures with the 365 μm fibers compared to the 272 μm ones, these occurring at a larger bend radius, but this difference was not significant. Conclusion: TFL appears to be a safer laser regarding the risk of fiber fracture than Ho:YAG when used with fibers in a deflected position.

Keywords: Ho:YAG laser; thulium fiber laser; laser fiber; lithotripsy; urolithiasis; ureteroscopy

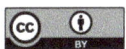

1. Introduction

Since its introduction in the 1990s, Ho:YAG laser has become the reference point for lasers for lithotripsy in urology because of its property to fragment all stone compositions, efficiencies and safety profiles [1–3]. Recently, a new laser has been released: the Super Pulsed Thulium Fiber Laser (TFL), with potential advantages over Ho:YAG laser such as higher ablation volumes during lithotripsy and production of thinner particles [4–8]. These two lasers use low hydroxyl silica optical fibers to transmit the laser beam to the stone [4,5,9,10]. During laser lithotripsy with flexible ureteroscopy (f-URS), laser fiber rupture may occur especially for lower pole stones treatment, resulting in working channel perforation and subsequent endoscope repair. Some studies reported risk factors of laser fiber fracture with Ho:YAG laser while bending: the diameter of the bend and high pulse energy [11,12]. While Ho:YAG laser and TFL are currently used for lithotripsy during f-URS, there is a lack of comparative study regarding the risk of laser fiber fracture during laser activation in a deflected position. Thus, we aimed to compare the risk of laser fiber fracture between Ho:YAG laser and TFL with different laser fiber diameters, laser settings, and fiber bending radii.

2. Materials and Methods

2.1. Laser Fibers

Single use laser fibers of a unique manufacturer (Rocamed, Monaco) with core diameters of 200, 272, and 365 µm were used for both laser systems to avoid any confusion due to a variability in laser fibers characteristics. Additionally, 150 µm laser fibers were also tested with the TFL only.

2.2. Laser Systems

A 50 W Super Pulsed TFL generator (IPG Photonics, Fryazino, Russia) with a wavelength of 1940 nm was compared to a 30 W Ho:YAG laser (MH01-ROCA FTS-30W, Rocamed, Monaco) with a wavelength of 2120 nm. A total of 13 different laser settings were tested for the Ho:YAG laser: 6 fragmentation settings with a short pulse duration, and 7 dusting settings with a long pulse duration. A total of 33 different laser settings were tested for the TFL. Since TFL offers lower energies and higher frequencies than current Ho:YAG lasers, we aimed to evaluate these specificities. Three laser settings were common to both lasers: 0.5 J × 12 Hz, 0.8 J × 8 Hz, 2 J × 3 Hz. All laser settings tested are presented in Table 1.

Table 1. (**A**): TFL laser settings; (**B**): Ho:YAG laser settings.

A. TFL Settings			
	6 W	25 W	50 W
Fine dusting (peak power = 125 W)			
0.025 J	240 Hz	1000 Hz	2000 Hz
0.05 J	120 Hz	500 Hz	1000 Hz
0.1 J	60 Hz	250 Hz	500 Hz
0.15 J	40 Hz	167 Hz	333 Hz
Dusting (peak power = 125 W)			
0.2 J	30 Hz	125 Hz	250 Hz
0.5 J	12 Hz	50 Hz	100 Hz
0.8 J	7.5 Hz	31.3 Hz	62.5 Hz
Fragmentation (peak power = 500 W)			
1 J	6 Hz	25 Hz	50 Hz
2 J	3 Hz	12.5 Hz	25 Hz
4 J	1.5 Hz	6.3 Hz	12.5 Hz
6 J	1 Hz	4.2 Hz	8.3 Hz
B. Ho:YAG Laser Settings			
Dusting (long pulse)			
0.2 J	25 Hz		
0.5 J	3 Hz	12 Hz	15 Hz
0.8 J	3 Hz	8 Hz	15 Hz
Fragmentation (short pulse)			
1 J	3 Hz	5 Hz	15 Hz
2 J	3 Hz	8 Hz	12 Hz

2.3. Experimental Setup

The laser fibers were supported by soft silicone tubes, secured by plastic screws (to hold the fibers without causing damage). Failure threshold testing was done by bending fibers to 180° with an initial radius of 1 cm, Figure 1A,B. In total, five different increasingly smaller bend radii were tested: 1, 0.9, 0.75, 0.6, and 0.45 cm. The choice of the minimal bending radius (0.45 cm) was based on the fact that we measured the most acute angle over several cases that a flexible ureteroscope might deflect for lower pole lithotripsy in difficult anatomical situations. Subsequent radii were randomly chosen to test wider values mimicking calices easier to navigate through. The laser was activated continuously for 5 min or until fiber fracture. Each measurement was performed ten times.

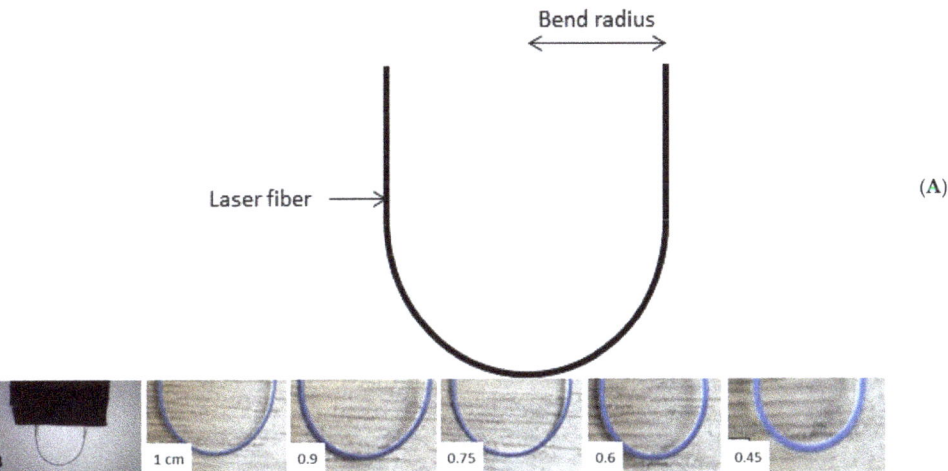

Figure 1. (**A**) Fiber bending radius, (**B**) Fiber bending radii tested.

2.4. Statistical Analyses

The Mann–Whitney test was used for comparisons between groups. All tests were conducted using the R Software, version 4.0.3. A *p*-value of 0.05 or less was considered significant.

3. Results

We did not report mechanical failure by bending the fibers alone. All fractures occurred after laser energy application.

3.1. Ho:YAG Laser

3.1.1. Dusting Settings

For the 200 µm fibers, the fracture rate was 50% at bending radius ≤0.6 cm, while none broke at radius ≥0.75 cm. For the 272 and 365 µm fiber diameters, fractures occurred only with a bending radius of 0.45 cm. A total of 20% of the 272 µm and 30% of the 365 µm fibers broke at a bend radius of 0.45 cm, Figure 2.

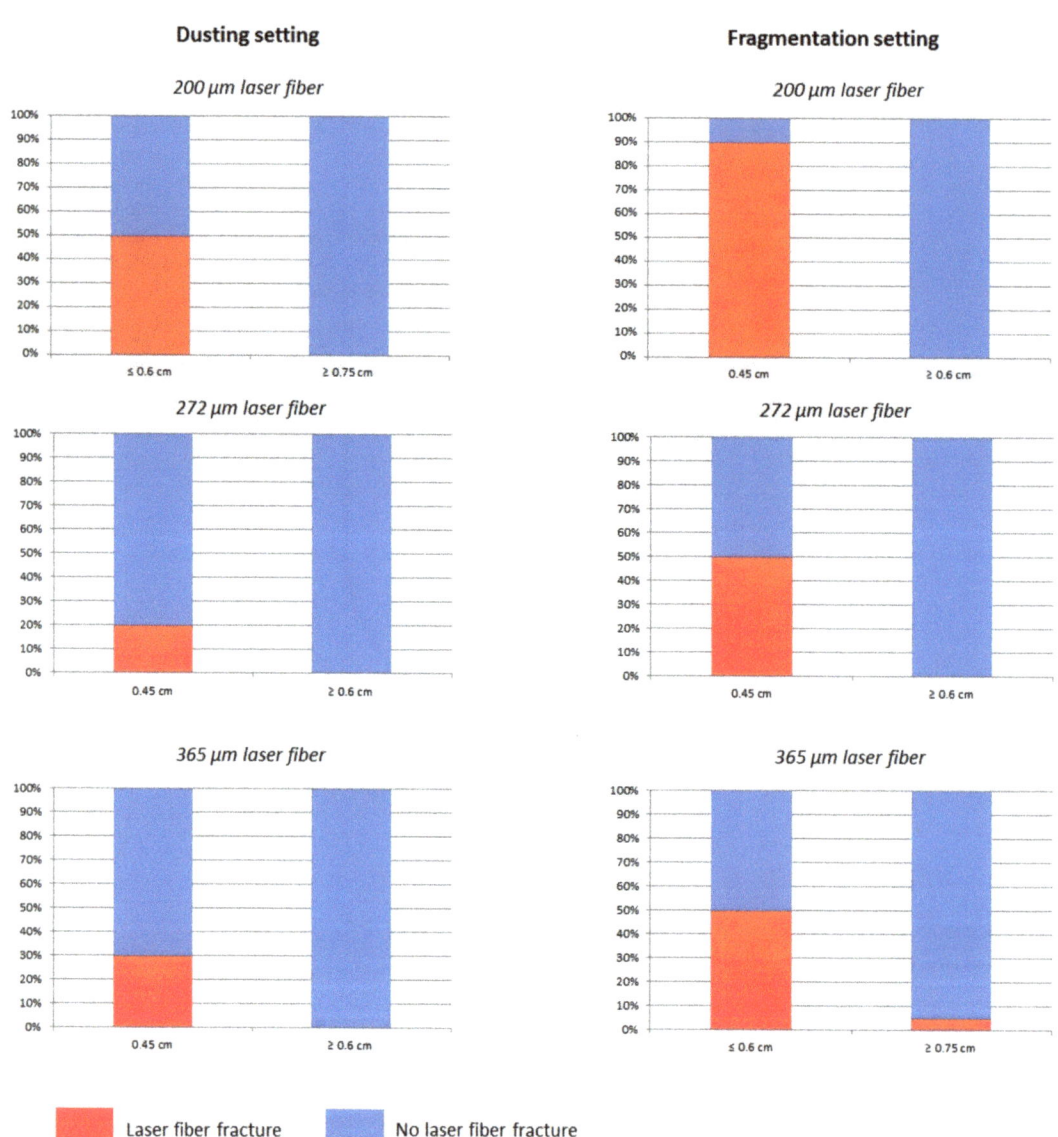

Figure 2. Proportion of fiber failures with Ho:YAG laser according to laser setting, fiber diameter, bending radius.

3.1.2. Fragmentation Settings

Of the 200 and 272 μm fibers, there was no fracture for a bend radius ≥0.6 cm. While 90% of the 200 μm fibers broke at a radius of 0.45 cm, 50% of the 272 μm did. The 365 μm fibers broke more frequently at ≤0.75 cm. A total of 5% and 50% of 365 μm laser fibers broke with a bending radius of ≥0.75 and ≤0.6 cm, respectively, Figure 2.

3.1.3. Identification of Risk Factors of Fiber Failure

Short pulse and high energy were significant risk factors of fiber fracture for the 365 μm fibers ($p = 0.041$), but not for the 200 and 272 μm fibers ($p = 1$ and $p = 0.43$, respectively). High frequency was not a risk factor of fiber fracture for all fiber core diameters.

Fiber diameter also seemed to be a risk factor of fracture. The 200 µm fibers broke more frequently than the 272 and 365 µm ones ($p = 0.039$). There was a trend for a higher number of fractures with the 365 µm fibers compared to the 272 µm ones, these occurring at a larger bend radius, but this difference was not significant.

3.2. TFL

Irrespective of the laser fiber diameter, laser settings, and bending radius, no fiber fracture occurred with the TFL.

3.3. Ho:YAG versus TFL

Irrespective of the laser settings, the fiber diameter and the bend radius, there was a significant risk of fiber fracture with the Ho:YAG laser compared to the TFL.

4. Discussion

The current study demonstrated a significant risk of fiber fracture with the Ho:YAG laser compared to the TFL in a deflected position. This result is of importance because nowadays f-URS has become a modality of choice for the treatment of kidney stones [13]. While Ho:YAG laser is currently the gold standard for lithotripsy during f-URS, TFL appears as an efficient alternative [14]. For both lasers, the laser energy is delivered to the target through a low hydroxyl silica fiber [9]. This laser fiber consists of a silica core through which the laser energy is transmitted. This core is surrounded by a layer called cladding that is essential for the efficient delivery of laser energy. This cladding is made of similar material to the core but has a different refractive index. Thus, the laser beam is reflected at the cladding–core interface. This process is called total internal reflection [9,10]. The most external part of the fiber is called jacket and encases the core and cladding. Its function is to protect the glass components of the fiber. When the fiber is bent, such as in lower pole stone treatment during f-URS, a small amount energy may leave the core to the cladding, and subsequently leak into the jacket. This condition represents a loss of total internal reflection of the laser energy, and once energy leaks into the jacket, fiber failure can occur due to thermal breakdown [15–17]. Prior studies demonstrated that the fibers do not fail with mechanical stress alone but rather fail when the laser is activated with the fiber in a deflected position. Consequences of such fiber failures are working channel perforations during laser activation, which represents an important cause of f-URS damage [18]. Several studies focused on the risk factors of fiber fracture in a deflected position with Ho:YAG laser [11,12,19–23]. They reported contradictory results regarding the influence of fiber diameter, bend radius, laser settings, and even for a same type of fiber from a specific manufacturer [12,20–22]. For example, while some authors reported that medium core fibers were prone to higher rates of failure than small core fibers, other studies did not document a correlation between increasing fiber diameter and fracture [11,20]. However, all the studies found that the resistance to fracture varies greatly among fiber manufacturers [12,20–22].

Similarly to Mues et al., we did not report mechanical failure by bending the fibers alone [21]. This means that failure is the consequence of loss of total internal reflection during laser activation in a bent fiber.

4.1. Ho:YAG Laser

The current study found that small core fibers (200 µm) were prone to a higher rate of fracture and failed at a larger bend radius ($\leq$0.6 cm) than 272 and 365 µm fibers in dusting setting (0.45 cm only). Surprisingly, no 200 µm fiber failure occurred at a bend radius $\geq$0.6 cm in fragmentation setting, but there was a higher proportion of fractures than in dusting setting (90% versus 50%, respectively). Thus, we found that small core fibers failed significantly more often than the 272 and 365 µm ones. These results are consistent with the report by Mues et al., and may be explained by the beam profile of the Ho:YAG laser [21]. Indeed, the Ho:YAG laser beam does not couple small core fibers

(<200 µm), and the risk may be overfilling the fiber core and leak laser energy to the fiber cladding, which can damage the fiber [4,5,24,25]. Thus, the use of small core fibers require the funneling of laser beam. As consequence, Ho:YAG laser is typically limited to larger fiber diameters (270–500 µm).

For the 272 and 365 µm fibers, we found similar results than Haddad et al., the 272 µm fibers failed at a smaller diameter than the 365 µm in fragmentation setting, but not in dusting setting.

Although 200 µm fibers are more flexible and may be more suitable for the treatment of lower pole stones during f-URS, they are more prone to failure when lasering. Thus, 272 µm core fibers seem a safer option for lower pole f-URS with Ho:YAG laser.

Finally, similarly to Knudsen et al., we found that the tightness of the fiber bend radius increases the risk of fiber failure as well as pulse energy for the 365 µm only [12]. This means that for a fixed bending radius, if the pulse energy increases, the amount of energy leaking the core to the cladding increases, and thus the risk of fiber fracture. On the contrary, Lusch et al. reported a trend for less fiber fracture at long pulse mode, high energy, low frequency in the small core fibers (200, 272/273 µm). Contrary to Vassar et al., we did not report an increase failure rate when the laser pulse energy increases with 272 µm fibers compared to the 365 µm [26].

4.2. TFL

Until now, no study has evaluated the risk of laser fiber fracture with the TFL. We found that, irrespective of the laser fiber diameter, laser settings, and bending radius, no fiber fracture occurred. These results may be explained by the beam profile and the peak power of the TFL. Contrary to the solid state Ho:YAG laser, the laser beam of the TFL originates within a small (18–25 µm) core of the thulium-doped silica optical fiber, which is about 100 times smaller in diameter than Ho:YAG laser. Furthermore, the TFL provides a near single mode Gaussian spatial beam profile, more uniform and symmetrical than the multimodal beam produced by the Ho:YAG laser [24]. Thus, even thinner laser fibers (150 µm) can be used with TFL. As consequence, total internal reflection may be respected in all fiber core diameters, with no leakage of energy through the cladding and jacket, which reduce the risk of fiber fracture. Moreover, peak power may also explain the absence of fracture with TFL. Indeed, the differences in fiber fracture rates between the two lasers systems may be explained by the constant higher peak power with the Ho:YAG laser compared to the TFL, regardless of the laser settings [27]. While peak power is directly correlated to the energy level with Ho:YAG laser and decreases with increased pulse duration, this remains constant with TFL. Furthermore, the pulse shape is also different with a flat and uniform shape for the TFL and a spike with an overshoot for the Ho:YAG laser [27]. Thus, the treatment of lower pole stone with TFL may be safer than with Ho:YAG laser, regardless of fiber diameter, bend radius, and laser settings.

Our study has several limitations, including the use of laser fibers from a unique manufacturer. However, by using exactly the same laser fiber manufacturer, it was possible to show the differences between both laser technologies, without risking the additional bias that using laser fibers from different origins might introduce. Yet, since great differences regarding size, flexibility, and resistance to fracture with bending among manufacturers exist, more optical fibers should be tested to ascertain our results with TFL. Although, laser fiber manufacturers provide short term minimum bending radius, we did not respect them in our tests since it is not possible to respect these minimal values in real conditions, especially in a difficult lower calyx access. Indeed, short term minimum bending radii were $\geq$13 mm, $\geq$17 mm, and $\geq$21 mm for the 200, 272, and 365 µm laser fibers tested, respectively. Another limitation was the absence of power transmission measurement. With transmission values, a quantitative correlation of core diameter, bending radius and losses might be possible. Lastly, laser activation duration was fixed at 5 min or until fiber fracture, which has resulted in different total energies delivered between powers tested.

However, this might affect the results with Ho:YAG laser only, since no fiber fracture occurred with TFL.

5. Conclusions

The is the first study comparing the risk of fiber fracture with different laser fiber diameters, laser settings, and fiber bending radii between the Ho:YAG laser and TFL. While fiber failures occurred with all fiber diameters with Ho:YAG laser, none was reported with TFL. Further studies testing fibers from different manufacturers are needed to ascertain these results.

Author Contributions: Conceptualization, S.D.; data curation, S.D. and O.T.; formal analysis, S.D., P.C. and F.P.; investigation, S.D., P.C. and F.P.; methodology, S.D and F.P.; project administration, S.D.; resources, S.D.; validation, S.D.; writing—original draft, A.U./S.D.; writing—review and editing, A.U., S.D., P.C. and F.P., M.H., L.B. and O.T. All authors have read and agreed to the published version of the manuscript.

Funding: This research received no external funding.

Institutional Review Board Statement: Not applicable.

Informed Consent Statement: Not applicable.

Data Availability Statement: Data are available by contacting authors.

Conflicts of Interest: Olivier Traxer is a consultant for: Boston Scientific, Coloplast, EMS, IPG Medical, Olympus, Rocamed. Audrey Uzan, Paul Chiron, Frédéric Panthier, Mattieu Haddad, Laurent Berthe, and Steeve Doizi have no conflict of interest to declare.

References

1. Johnson, D.E.; Cromeens, D.M.; Price, R.E. Use of the holmium:YAG laser in urology. *Lasers Surg. Med.* **1992**, *12*, 353–363. [CrossRef]
2. Herrmann, T.R.; Liatsikos, E.N.; Nagele, U.; Traxer, O.; Merseburger, A.S. EAU Guidelines on Laser Technologies. *Eur. Urol.* **2012**, *61*, 783–795. [CrossRef]
3. Sayer, J.; Johnson, D.E.; Price, R.E.; Cromeens, D.M. Endoscopic laser fragmentation of ureteral calculi using the holmium:YAG. *Proc. SPIE* **1993**, *1879*, 143–148. [CrossRef]
4. Fried, N.M. Recent advances in infrared laser lithotripsy [Invited]. *Biomed. Opt. Express* **2018**, *9*, 4552–4568. [CrossRef] [PubMed]
5. Fried, N.M.; Irby, P.B. Advances in laser technology and fibre-optic delivery systems in lithotripsy. *Nat. Rev. Urol.* **2018**, *15*, 563–573. [CrossRef] [PubMed]
6. Keller, E.X.; De Coninck, V.; Doizi, S.; Daudon, M.; Traxer, O. Thulium fiber laser: Ready to dust all urinary stone composition types? *World J. Urol.* **2021**, *39*, 1693–1698. [CrossRef]
7. Panthier, F.; Doizi, S.; Lapouge, P.; Chaussain, C.; Kogane, N.; Berthe, L.; Traxer, O. Comparison of the ablation rates, fissures and fragments produced with 150 microm and 272 microm laser fibers with superpulsed thulium fiber laser: An in vitro study. *World J. Urol.* **2021**, *39*, 1683–1691. [CrossRef] [PubMed]
8. Traxer, O.; Keller, E.X. Thulium fiber laser: The new player for kidney stone treatment? A comparison with Holmium:YAG laser. *World J. Urol.* **2020**, *38*, 1883–1894. [CrossRef] [PubMed]
9. Nazif, O.A.; Teichman, J.M.; Glickman, R.D.; Welch, A.J. Review of Laser Fibers: A Practical Guide for Urologists. *J. Endourol.* **2004**, *18*, 818–829. [CrossRef]
10. Knudsen, B.E. Laser Fibers for Holmium:YAG Lithotripsy: What Is Important and What Is New. *Urol. Clin. N. Am.* **2019**, *46*, 185–191. [CrossRef]
11. Haddad, M.; Emiliani, E.; Rouchausse, Y.; Coste, F.; Doizi, S.; Berthe, L.; Butticè, S.; Somani, B.K.; Traxer, O. Impact of the Curve Diameter and Laser Settings on Laser Fiber Fracture. *J. Endourol.* **2017**, *31*, 918–921. [CrossRef] [PubMed]
12. Knudsen, B.E.; Glickman, R.D.; Stallman, K.J.; Maswadi, S.; Chew, B.H.; Beiko, D.T.; Denstedt, J.D.; Teichman, J.M. Performance and Safety of Holmium:YAG Laser Optical Fibers. *J. Endourol.* **2005**, *19*, 1092–1097. [CrossRef] [PubMed]
13. Türk, C.; Knoll, T.; Petrik, A.; Sarica, K.; Skolarikos, A.; Straub, M.; Seitz, C. EAU Guidelines on Urolithiasis. *Eur. Urol.* **2021**. Available online: https://uroweb.org/guideline/urolithiasis/ (accessed on 10 May 2021).
14. Enikeev, D.; Traxer, O.; Taratkin, M.; Okhunov, Z.; Shariat, S. A review of thulium-fiber laser in stone lithotripsy and soft tissue surgery. *Curr. Opin. Urol.* **2020**, *30*, 853–860. [CrossRef] [PubMed]
15. Lee, H.; Ryan, R.T.; Teichman, J.M.; Landman, J.; Clayman, R.V.; Milner, T.E.; Welch, A.J. Effect of lithotripsy on holmium:YAG optical beam profile. *J. Endourol.* **2003**, *17*, 63–67. [CrossRef]
16. Marks, A.J.; Teichman, J.M.H. Lasers in clinical urology: State of the art and new horizons. *World J. Urol.* **2007**, *25*, 227–233. [CrossRef]

17. Heckscher, D.; Zeng, J.; Samolis, P.; Sander, M.Y.; Wason, S.E.L.; Wang, D.S. The Effect of Holmium Laser Fiber Bending Radius on Power Delivery During Flexible Ureteroscopy. *J. Endourol.* **2020**, *34*, 682–686. [CrossRef]
18. Afane, J.S.; Olweny, E.O.; Bercowsky, E.; Sundaram, C.P.; Dunn, M.D.; Shalhav, A.L.; McDougall, E.M.; Clayman, R.V. Flexible ureteroscopes: A single center evaluation of the durability and function of the new endoscopes smaller than 9Fr. *J. Urol.* **2000**, *164*, 1164–1168. [CrossRef]
19. Bourdoumis, A.; Christopoulos, P.; Raj, N.; Fedder, A.; Buchholz, N. A Comparative in Vitro Study of Power Output Deterioration over Time Between Ho:YAG Laser Fibers from Different Manufacturers as a Function of Deflection and Power Input. *Curr. Urol.* **2016**, *9*, 12–18. [CrossRef]
20. Akar, E.C.; Knudsen, B.E. Evaluation of 16 New Holmium: Yttrium-Aluminum-Garnet Laser Optical Fibers for Ureteroscopy. *Urology* **2015**, *86*, 230–235. [CrossRef] [PubMed]
21. Mues, A.C.; Teichman, J.M.; Knudsen, B.E. Evaluation of 24 Holmium:YAG Laser Optical Fibers for Flexible Ureteroscopy. *J. Urol.* **2009**, *182*, 348–354. [CrossRef] [PubMed]
22. Lusch, A.; Heidari, E.; Okhunov, Z.; Osann, K.; Landman, J. Evaluation of Contemporary Holmium Laser Fibers for Performance Characteristics. *J. Endourol.* **2016**, *30*, 567–573. [CrossRef]
23. Khemees, T.A.; Shore, D.M.; Antiporda, M.; Teichman, J.M.; Knudsen, B.E. Evaluation of a new 240-mum single-use holmium:YAG optical fiber for flexible ureteroscopy. *J. Endourol.* **2013**, *27*, 475–479. [CrossRef]
24. Griffin, S. Fiber optics for destroying kidney stones. *Biophotonics Int.* **2004**, *11*, 44–47.
25. Hutchens, T.C.; Gonzalez, D.A.; Irby, P.B.; Fried, N.M. Fiber optic muzzle brake tip for reducing fiber burnback and stone retropulsion during thulium fiber laser lithotripsy. *J. Biomed. Opt.* **2017**, *22*, 018001. [CrossRef]
26. Vassar, G.J.; Teichman, J.M.; Glickman, R.D. Holmium:YAG Lithotripsy Efficiency Varies with Energy Density. *J. Urol.* **1998**, *160*, 471–476. [CrossRef]
27. Ventimiglia, E.; Doizi, S.; Kovalenko, A.; Andreeva, V.; Traxer, O. Effect of temporal pulse shape on urinary stone phantom retropulsion rate and ablation efficiency using holmium:YAG and super-pulse thulium fibre lasers. *BJU Int.* **2020**, *126*, 159–167. [CrossRef]

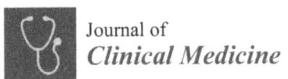

Article

Global Variations in the Mineral Content of Bottled Still and Sparkling Water and a Description of the Possible Impact on Nephrological and Urological Diseases

Simone J. M. Stoots [1,*], Guido M. Kamphuis [1], Rob Geraghty [2], Liffert Vogt [3], Michaël M. E. L. Henderickx [1], B. M. Zeeshan Hameed [4], Sufyan Ibrahim [4], Amelia Pietropaolo [5], Enakshee Jamnadass [5], Sahar M. Aljumaiah [6], Saeed B. Hamri [6], Eugenio Ventimiglia [7], Olivier Traxer [8], Vineet Gauhar [9], Etienne X. Keller [10], Vincent De Coninck [11], Otas Durutovic [12], Nariman K. Gadzhiev [13], Laurian B. Dragos [14], Tarik Emre Sener [15], Nick Rukin [16], Michele Talso [17], Panagiotis Kallidonis [18], Esteban Emiliani [19], Ewa Bres-Niewada [20], Kymora B. Scotland [21], Naeem Bhojani [22], Athanasios Vagionis [18], Angela Piccirilli [19] and Bhaskar K. Somani [5]

Citation: Stoots, S.J.M.; Kamphuis, G.M.; Geraghty, R.; Vogt, L.; Henderickx, M.M.E.L.; Hameed, B.M.Z.; Ibrahim, S.; Pietropaolo, A.; Jamnadass, E.; Aljumaiah, S.M.; et al. Global Variations in the Mineral Content of Bottled Still and Sparkling Water and a Description of the Possible Impact on Nephrological and Urological Diseases. *J. Clin. Med.* 2021, *10*, 2807. https://doi.org/10.3390/jcm10132807

Academic Editors: Javier Donate-Correa and San-e Ishikawa

Received: 25 May 2021
Accepted: 15 June 2021
Published: 27 June 2021

Publisher's Note: MDPI stays neutral with regard to jurisdictional claims in published maps and institutional affiliations.

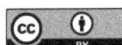

Copyright: © 2021 by the authors. Licensee MDPI, Basel, Switzerland. This article is an open access article distributed under the terms and conditions of the Creative Commons Attribution (CC BY) license (https://creativecommons.org/licenses/by/4.0/).

1. Department of Urology, Amsterdam UMC, AMC, University of Amsterdam, 1105 Amsterdam, The Netherlands; g.m.kamphuis@amsterdamumc.nl (G.M.K.); m.m.henderickx@amsterdamumc.nl (M.M.E.L.H.)
2. Department of Urology, Freeman Hospital, Newcastle NE7 7DN, UK; robgeraghty@btinternet.com
3. Department of Internal Medicine, Section Nephrology, Amsterdam UMC, AMC, University of Amsterdam, 1105 Amsterdam, The Netherlands; l.vogt@amsterdamumc.nl
4. Department of Urology, Kasturba Medical College and Hospital, Manipal Academy of Higher Education, Manipal, Karnataka 576104, India; zeeshanhameedbm@gmail.com (B.M.Z.H.); sufyan.ibrahim2@gmail.com (S.I.)
5. Department of Urology, University Hospital Southampton NHS Trust, Southampton SO16 6YD, UK; amelia.pietropaolo@uhs.nhs.uk (A.P.); enakshee@gmail.com (E.J.); bhaskarsomani@yahoo.com (B.K.S.)
6. Department of Urology, Ministry of the National Guard—Health Affairs, Riyadh 11426, Saudi Arabia; jumaiahsa@gmail.com (S.M.A.); sbinhamri@gmail.com (S.B.H.)
7. Division of Experimental Oncology/Unit of Urology, IRCCS Ospedale, Urological Research Institute, San Raffaele, 20132 Milan, Italy; eugenio.ventimiglia@gmail.com
8. Department of Urology, Sorbonne University, GRC #20 urolithiasis, 75006 Paris, France; traxer.olivier@gmail.com
9. Department of Urology, Ng Teng Fong General Hospital, Singapore 609606, Singapore; vineetgaauhaar@gmail.com
10. Department of Urology, University Hospital Zurich, University of Zurich, 8091 Zurich, Switzerland; etienne.xavier.keller@gmail.com
11. Department of Urology, AZ Klina, 2930 Brasschaat, Belgium; vincent.de.coninck@klina.be
12. Department of Urology, University Clinical Center of Serbia, University of Belgrade, 11000 Belgrade, Serbia; odurutovic@gmail.com
13. Department of Urology, Saint-Petersburg State University Hospital, 197022 Saint Petersburg, Russia; nariman.gadjiev@gmail.com
14. Department of Urology, Addenbrooke's Hospital, Hills Road, Cambridge CB2 0QQ, UK; lauriandragos@yahoo.com
15. Department of Urology, Marmara University Hospital, Marmara University School of Medicine, Istanbul 34854, Turkey; dr.emresener@gmail.com
16. Department of Urology, Redcliff Hospital, Brisbane QLD 4012, Australia; nickrukin@hotmail.com
17. Department of Urology, ASST Fatebenefratelli-Sacco, Luigi Sacco University Hospital, 20157 Milan, Italy; michele.talso@gmail.com
18. Department of Urology, University of Patras, 26504 Patras, Greece; pkallidonis@yahoo.com (P.K.); thanos_vagionis@hotmail.gr (A.V.)
19. Department of Urology, Fundació Puigvert, Autonomous University of Barcelona, 08025 Barcelona, Spain; emiliani@gmail.com (E.E.); angelapiccirilli@yahoo.it (A.P.)
20. Department of Urology, Medical University of Warsaw, 02-091 Warsaw, Poland; ewa.bres@gmail.com
21. Department of Urology, University of California Los Angeles (UCLA), Los Angeles, CA 90095, USA; kscotland@mednet.ucla.edu
22. Department of Urology, University of Montreal, Montreal, QC H2X 0A9, Canada; naeem.bhojani@gmail.com
* Correspondence: s.j.stoots@amsterdamumc.nl

Abstract: Kidney stone disease (KSD) is a complex disease. Besides the high risk of recurrence, its association with systemic disorders contributes to the burden of disease. Sufficient water intake is crucial for prevention of KSD, however, the mineral content of water might influence stone formation, bone health and cardiovascular (CVD) risk. This study aims to analyse the variations in mineral content of bottled drinking water worldwide to evaluate the differences and describes the possible impact on nephrological and urological diseases. The information regarding mineral composition (mg/L) on calcium, bicarbonate, magnesium, sodium and sulphates was read from the ingredients label on water bottles by visiting the supermarket or consulting the online shop. The bottled waters in two main supermarkets in 21 countries were included. The evaluation shows that on a global level the mineral composition of bottled drinkable water varies enormously. Median bicarbonate levels varied by factors of 12.6 and 57.3 for still and sparkling water, respectively. Median calcium levels varied by factors of 18.7 and 7.4 for still and sparkling water, respectively. As the mineral content of bottled drinking water varies enormously worldwide and mineral intake through water might influence stone formation, bone health and CVD risk, urologists and nephrologists should counsel their patients on an individual level regarding water intake.

Keywords: kidney stone disease; mineral water; mineral composition; drinking water; still water; sparkling water

1. Introduction

Kidney stone disease (KSD), a condition characterized by the formation of crystals within the urinary tract, is a prevalent disease worldwide. Especially in Western countries, hypothetically due to an increase in obesity, diabetes and improved diagnostics, the estimated lifetime prevalence has risen to 14% [1-3]. Currently, prevalence rates range from 7-13% in The United States, 5-14% in Europe and 1-5% in Asia [3]. Besides a high risk of recurrence of 53% at 5 years, another factor contributing to the burden of disease is its association with systemic disorders like coronary heart disease, hypertension, diabetes type 2 and osteoporosis. [4-8].

Although KSD has a complex pathophysiology with a multifactorial aetiology, it is important to understand the various processes leading to stone formation to be able to develop a preventive strategy, to reduce precipitation of crystal-forming substances leading to stone formation. The most recognized general intervention regarding primary prevention for stone formation in patients with KSD, regardless of stone composition, is sufficient fluid intake [9,10]. By increasing the urinary output to at least 2 L/day, dilution of stone forming salts occurs, reducing urinary supersaturation. At the same time, stagnation of urine within the urinary tract, a mechanical risk factor for stone formation, is less likely to occur with sufficient diuresis [11,12].

Although the benefit of water therapy was primarily recognized for the prevention of urolithiasis, it seems to be beneficial in other renal diseases as well. A higher water intake is associated with a reduction in cyst growth rate in autosomal dominant polycystic kidney disease (ADPKD) and seems to protect against chronic kidney disease (CKD), and might even slow the progression of CKD [13].

Over time, scientists have investigated the impact of the mineral content of drinking water on our health. Mineral water rich in calcium and bicarbonate for example, provide for an increase in bone mineral density and a decrease in bone resorption [14,15]. Furthermore, magnesium levels in drinking water seem to be inversely related to the risk of death due to coronary heart disease [16].

Regarding KSD, several minerals have been designated as promotors or inhibitors of stone formation. High urinary excretion of calcium, oxalate and uric acid are well known promoters. On the contrary, urinary citrate, potassium and bicarbonate might be protective factors regarding stone formation [17-19]. By analysing 24 h urine samples, which is recommended for high-risk stone formers, urine chemistry may reveal such metabolic abnormalities [20].

As sufficient fluid intake seems to be crucial in the prevention of KSD, the question arises as to what fluids to drink. Beverages like soda, lemonade and fruit juices are not recommended due to their high levels of fructose. Although coffee, tea, wine and beer seem to lower the risk for stone formation [21], physicians generally advise their patients to drink water as it is free from caffeine, alcohol and calories. However, we must realize that drinking water may also contain certain minerals that could lead to a rise of urinary stone promotors and inhibitors. Earlier research performed in France, Spain and the USA has already shown a variation in the mineral content of tap and bottled water nationwide [22–24]. European studies showed that the mineral composition of commercially available bottled drinking water across Europe varies enormously [25,26]. Possibly, drinking water with certain characteristics could increase stone risk where others might be better in the inhibition of stone formation.

As the consumption of bottled water is increasing worldwide and is not subject to such strict regulations compared to tap water, it is important to gain insight into mineral composition and the possible impact on our health. Therefore, this study aims to analyse the variations in mineral content of bottled 'still' and bottled 'sparkling or carbonated' water across different manufacturers and countries worldwide to evaluate the differences globally. This study also aims to describe the possible consequences of the mineral composition of drinking water on our general health, with a focus on nephrological and urological diseases.

2. Materials and Methods

This descriptive, multi-continental study was conducted to enhance the understanding of the variabilities of mineral content of commercially available bottled drinking water worldwide. The mineral content of bottled still water and bottled sparkling or carbonated water across different manufacturers was analysed globally. For data collection, the information regarding mineral composition was read from the manufacturers' ingredient label on water bottles which were commercially available in the two main supermarket chains of each country. As an alternative, the online shop of the supermarket could be used. Minerals of interest were bicarbonate, calcium, magnesium, potassium, sodium and sulphates. All data were obtained in milligrams per litre (mg/L) or otherwise converted to mg/L.

The study was conducted in 21 countries worldwide including: Australia, Belgium, Brazil, Canada, France, Germany, Greece, India, Italy, The Netherlands, Poland, Romania, Russia, Saudi Arabia, Serbia, Singapore, Spain, Switzerland, Turkey, The United Kingdom and The United States.

For statistical analysis, the software of SPSS, version 26 (IBM Corp., Armonk, NY, USA), was used. A check for normality showed that the data were not normally distributed, therefore they were treated as non-parametric data. Descriptive statistics and simple boxplots were used to graphically show the distributional features of the data. To improve the visual representation of the data, some extreme values were excluded from the boxplots. The data are available as supplement to the figures.

3. Results

For bottled still water, 316 different commercial water brands were analysed. 29 brands (Acqua Panna, Albert Heijn, Aqua, Aquarel, Bar le Duc, Bleu, Cactus, Cano, Chaudfontaine, Contrex, Dassani, Evian, Fiji, Glaceau Smart water, Harrogate, Hépar, Ice Mountain, Life, Meadows, Montcalm, Nestlé PureLife, pH Balancer, pH Infinity, San Benedetto, Solar de Cabras, Vittel, Volvic, Voss, Zagori) were available in up to 11 countries. Table 1 shows the mineral composition (mg/L) of bottled still water by country expressed as median (IQR). Globally, the median mineral content of still water per mineral varies greatly. Median bicarbonate levels for example vary by a factor of 12.6. Calcium levels vary by a factor of 18.7. Median potassium levels did not vary a lot, ranging from 0.7 mg/L to 2.8 mg/L.

Table 1. The mineral composition (mg/L) of bottled still water expressed as median (IQR).

Country	Mineral Composition (mg/L)					
	Bicarbonate	Calcium	Magnesium	Potassium	Sodium	Sulphates
Australia	130.00 (34.00–258.00)	18.00 (6.40–31.95)	3.95 (0.525–16.50)	0.70 (0.17–1.60)	6.60 (3.79–12.00)	6.55 (3.40–14.00)
Belgium	301.00 (180.00–360.00)	66.80 (16.50–101.00)	18.00 (1.80–26.00)	2.00 (0.60–4.00)	8.50 (3.25–15.60)	18.00 (10.00–40.00)
Brazil	50.71 (13.20–95.49)	5.78 (3.43–13.30)	2.42 (1.55–4.71)	1.42 (1.22–4.00)	4.95 (3.34–13.93)	1.56 (0.93–2.95)
Canada	210.00 (35.00–330.00)	42.00 (7.00–73.00)	9.60 (2.50–25.15)	1.30 (1.00–3.00)	6.00 (2.48–13.00)	4.10 (1.50–12.55)
France	163.50 (127.00–372.00)	68.00 (19.00–468.00)	26.00 (8.00–56.00)	2.80 (1.60–4.00)	6.50 (3.00–11.60)	24.00 (8.10–1121)
Germany	270.00 (182.00–356.50)	94.00 (47.00–142.00)	25.25 (6.65–43.50)	1.75 (1.15–4.65)	14.40 (7.10–17.30)	39.55 (9.00–162.00)
Greece	244.00 (182.00–286.00)	79.65 (60.00–93.10)	7.00 (3.30–12.80)	0.79 (0.60–1.00)	4.90 (4.35–7.80)	9.15 (5.00–14.00)
India	158.50 (64.00–196.80)	17.00 (13.60–33.60)	9.65 (6.20–22.00)	2.60 (0.50–4.00)	7.45 (1.55–28.2)	6.00 (3.20–19.30)
Italy	106.00 (50.00–296.00)	32.20 (11.80–60.36)	4.90 (3.70–22.10)	0.80 (0.35–1.60)	2.20 (1.00–6.00)	8.60 (6.00–22.00)
The Netherlands	190.00 (106.00–305.00)	60.00 (15.00–80.00)	6.25 (2.46–18.00)	1.00 (0.60–3.30)	10.60 (4.80–36.20)	34.00 (10.00–40.00)
Poland	314.45 (223.40–512.45)	70.13 (43.85–111.20)	19.75 (9.92–28.55)	1.28 (0.89–2.50)	9.85 (7.28–11.05)	7.94 (0.00–36.25)
Romania	81.11 (28.00–192.03)	57.85 (43.50–62.77)	7.50 (2.21–20.60)	0.75 (0.40–1.70)	2.33 (0.93–12.74)	10.70 (2.10–19.29)
Russia	152.00 (45.00–258.00)	43.30 (21.20–70.60)	17.40 (6.22–21.40)	1.95 (1.03–5.00)	5.96 (4.10–9.29)	8.50 (6.12–31.00)
Saudi Arabia	25.00 (6.10–50.00)	21.50 (12.00–40.50)	4.70 (2.00–13.00)	1.00 (0.70–1.40)	5.00 (3.80–17.00)	21.80 (4.00–30.00)
Serbia	292.5 (106.00–400.80)	64.01 (33.82–79.90)	19.50 (6.50–34.00)	1.05 (0.59–2.96)	6.60 (2.10–11.50)	11.55 (7.15–23.00)
Singapore	125.00 (71.00–150.00)	30.50 (15.00–37.10)	3.20 (2.10–8.00)	2.15 (1.80–2.30)	2.80 (1.80–5.20)	6.00 (3.00–9.10)
Spain	199.30 (129.20–275.00)	50.79 (24.25–75.25)	11.50 (5.00–23.40)	1.45 (0.90–2.30)	9.00 (4.70–27.00)	14.40 (8.10–26.75)
Switzerland	252.00 (226.30–289.00)	108.00 (89.00–221.00)	24.00 (17.00–39.00)	1.80 (0.80–2.50)	5.00 (4.00–6.50)	170.00 (29.50–597.00)
Turkey	125.00 (71.00–150.00)	30.50 (15.00–37.10)	3.20 (2.10–8.00)	2.15 (1.80–2.30)	2.80 (1.80–5.20)	4.50 (2.90–8.60)
The United Kingdom	171.00 (74.00–240.00)	55.00 (12.00–59.00)	10.05 (3.50–19.00)	1.20 (1.00–2.50)	11.90 (7.03–15.00)	12.00 (9.00–14.00)
The United States	118.50 (76.00–155.00)	12.00 (8.70–26.20)	5.05 (2.10–8.05)	1.90 (1.50–4.90)	7.25 (6.15–11.55)	5.65 (3.80–10.00)

Figure 1A–F shows the distribution of the mineral composition (mg/L) of bottled still water worldwide.

Overall, for still water, bicarbonate levels ranged from 0 mg/L (Pureau—Australia, Speyside Glenlivet—Saudi Arabia, Solan de Cabras—Saudi Arabia, Voss—Saudi Arabia) to 2495 mg/L (Heppinger Extra Heil water—Germany) worldwide. Outliers and extreme values for bicarbonate which are excluded in Figure 1 are Sangemini (1010 mg/L), Piwniczanka (1260 mg/L), Zywiec Zdrój (1404 mg/L), Gerolsteiner (1816 mg/L), Staatl. Fachingen Still (1846 mg/L), Heppinger Extra Heil (2495 mg/L). Calcium levels ranged from 0 mg/L (Moores Ultra Pure—Australia) to 579 mg/L (Abdelbodner Cristal—Switzerland). Magnesium levels ranged from 0 mg/L (Moores Ultra Pure—Australia, E'stel—Australia) to 199 mg/L (Heppinger Extra Heil water—Germany). The outliers and extremes were

Piwniczanka (87 mg/L), Gerolsteiner (108 mg/L), Eptinger Still (117 mg/L), Abatilles (119 mg/L), Hépar (119 mg/L) and Heppinger Extra Heil (199 mg/L).

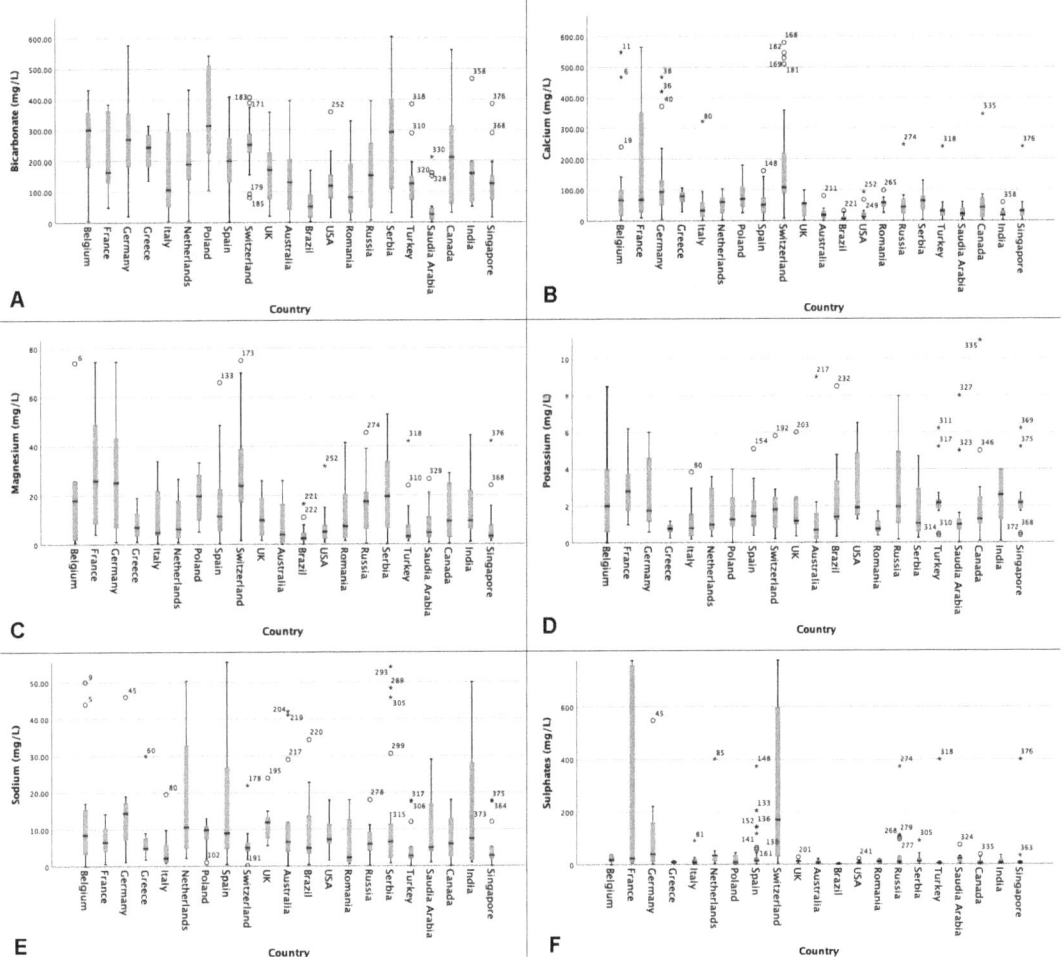

Figure 1. (A–F): The mineral composition of bottled still water (mg/L) per mineral by country. ° Outlier. * Extreme value.

Potassium levels ranged from 0 mg/L (Voss—Saudi Arabia/Australia, Spa Reine—Belgium, Żywiec Zdrój—Poland, Harrogate—Saudi Arabia, Dobrowinka—Poland, Contrex—Belgium, Aqua Nordic Naturelle—Germany) to 27.1 mg/L (Aqua Nordic Naturell—Germany). Outliers and extremes excluded in Figure 1 were Piwniczanka (13 mg/L), De L'Aubier (16 mg/L), Staatl. Fachingen Still (16 mg/L), Cristaline (18 mg/L), Heppinger Extra Heil (27 mg/L) and Aqua Nordic Naturelle (92 mg/L).

Sodium levels ranged from 0 mg/L (Jackson Springs—Canada, Dassani—Turkey/Saudi Arabia, Moores Ultra Pure—Australia, Albert Heijn—Belgium, Pureau—Australia) to 564 mg/L (Staatl. Fachingen Still—Germany). For sodium, many outliers and extreme values were identified. Excluded from Figure 1 are Contrex Still (59 mg/L), Aquavia (65 mg/L), Pine Cone Forest (86 mg/L), Perla Covasnei (90 mg/L), Ibira (91 mg/L), Carrefour (95 mg/L), Fontecelto (95 mg/L), Gerolsteiner (118 mg/L), Boni (125 mg/L),

Piwniczanka (133 mg/L), Zurzacher Naturelle (154 mg/L), Abatilles (200 mg/L), Saint-Justin (415 mg/L), Heppinger Extra Heil (481 mg/L) and Staatl. Fachingen (564 mg/L).

Sulphates levels ranged from 0 mg/L (Jackson Springs—Australia, Górska Natura—Poland, Dobrowinka—Poland, Żywiec Zdrój—Poland, Nałęczowianka—Poland, Aquarel Nestlé—Poland, Ordal—Belgium, Saint-Justin—Canada) to 190.4 mg/L (Buzias (light)—Romania). Outliers and extremes were Extaler Mineralqual Naturelle (900 mg/L), Carolinen Naturelle (950 mg/L), Contrex Still (1121 mg/L), and Hépar (1530 mg/L).

In total, 224 different commercial water brands were included for sparkling or carbonated water. Seventeen of them (Badoit, Bar le Duc, Cano, Chaudfontaine, Evian Blue, Gerolsteiner, Gerolsteiner Medium, Highland Spring, H-two-O, Nestlé PureLife, Oldenladia, Perrier, San Benedetto, San Pelligrino, Sourcy, Souroti, Voss) were available in up to 10 different countries. Table 2 shows the mineral composition (mg/L) of bottled sparkling or carbonated water by country expressed as median (IQR). As for still water, median levels of the mineral content of sparkling water vary greatly as well, with variations in median bicarbonate levels ranging from 22 mg/L to 1260 mg/L and median magnesium levels varying from 4 mg/L to 53 mg/L.

Table 2. The mineral composition (mg/L) of bottled sparkling water expressed as median (IQR).

Country	Mineral Composition (mg/L)					
	Bicarbonate	Calcium	Magnesium	Potassium	Sodium	Sulphates
Australia	233.00 (200.00–243.00)	37.75 (25.98–95.60)	19.00 (4.00–29.00)	1.00 (0.00–2.00)	7.00 (1.90–10.00)	16.00 (6.00–33.00)
Belgium	22.00 (180.00–317.00)	56.00 (13.50–151.50)	7.00 (2.00–18.00)	2.00 (1.00–5.00)	10.60 (9.00–33.30)	19.00 (8.00–33.00)
Brazil	102.84 (91.41–203.28)	17.14 (13.90–26.05)	4.00 (3.00–7.00)	1.00 (1.00–3.00)	11.80 (3.98–23.02)	6.00 (2.00–38.00)
Canada	176.60 (77.00–243.00)	51.00 (42.00–150.00)	16.00 (6.00–29.00)	2.00 (1.00–4.00)	10.00 (6.00–36.10)	25.00 (11.00–125.00)
France	1175.00 (710.00–1837.00)	151.50 (90.00–185.00)	15.00 (8.00–49.00)	34.00 (11.00–52.00)	210.00 (7.47–381.00)	30.00 (20.00–59.00)
Germany	253.00 (189.00–349.00)	67.50 (47.00–142.00)	23.00 (5.00–42.00)	2.00 (1.00–4.00)	15.80 (13.30–29.90)	36.00 (9.00–162.00)
Greece	344.15 (274.00–781.00)	87.20 (59.30–188.00)	24.00 (3.00–53.00)	0.00 (0.00–0.00)	6.02 (4.43–20.00)	11.00 (5.00–12.00)
India	243.00 (155.00–390.00)	94.30 (3.65–155.65)	8.00 (5.00–30.00)	2.00 (1.00–13.00)	20.00 (9.00–31.20)	33.00 (24.00–402.00)
Italy	212.55 (57.40–930.00)	43.50 (9.10–164.00)	13.00 (2.00–25.00)	1.00 (1.00–2.00)	3.07 (1.50–6.00)	6.00 (4.00–18.00)
The Netherlands	190.00 (170.00–360.00)	68.50 (40.90–101.50)	7.00 (3.00–18.00)	2.00 (1.00–3.00)	10.30 (6.00–30.60)	29.00 (9.00–37.00)
Poland	1260.00 (335.60–1550.00)	180.90 (97.80–301.00)	52.00 (13.00–153.00)	7.00 (2.00–49.00)	63.00 (4.59–118.00)	29.00 (27.00–32.00)
Romania	648.00 (244.00–1364.50)	104.00 (74.85–252.60)	34.00 (11.00–49.00)	7.00 (1.00–9.00)	51.40 (15.41–205.00)	1.00 (1.00–16.00)
Russia	218.50 (107.00–330.00)	40.20 (21.60–101.00)	19.00 (6.00–33.00)	4.00 (1.00–9.00)	10.41 (4.90–135.00)	10.00 (5.00–30.00)
Saudi Arabia	100.00 (0.00–744.00)	151.50 (22.00–182.00)	28.00 (4.00–54.00)	4.00 (1.00–11.00)	23.50 (9.60–122.00)	25.00 (5.00–35.00)
Serbia	1251.00 (423.00–2100.00)	80.00 (67.84–114.00)	43.00 (40.00–68.00)	19.00 (3.00–39.00)	200.70 (14.10–598.00)	39.00 (11.00–116.00)
Singapore	360.00 (205.00–1250.00)	37.10 (1.00–153.00)	30.00 (16.00–80.00)	11.00 (5.00–11.00)	120.50 (24.75–148.00)	28.00 (18.00–37.00)
Spain	287.00 (215.50–1935.50)	55.00 (32.00–86.80)	8.00 (4.00–31.00)	9.00 (3.00–49.00)	38.80 (7.55–835.50)	11.00 (7.00–48.00)

Table 2. Cont.

Country	Mineral Composition (mg/L)					
	Bicarbonate	Calcium	Magnesium	Potassium	Sodium	Sulphates
Switzerland	273.50 (243.50–360.50)	191.00 (97.70–330.00)	36.00 (22.00–52.00)	2.00 (1.00–3.00)	5.20 (4.00–7.00)	263.00 (55.00–885.00)
Turkey	360.00 (205.00–1250.00)	80.00 (37.10–153.00)	53.00 (21.00–94.00)	11.00 (6.00–28.00)	120.50 (6.50–128.00)	35.00 (14.00–38.00)
The United Kingdom	240.00 (215.00–245.00)	56.00 (55.00–104.00)	18.00 (10.00–19.00)	2.00 (1.00–2.00)	11.50 (7.47–24.00)	13.00 (9.00–28.00)
The United States	n.a.	25.95 (6.65–130.00)	4.00 (2.00–8.00)	2.00 (2.00–4.00)	8.30 (3.30–11.00)	20.00 (11.00–26.00)

Figure 2A–F shows the distribution of the mineral composition (mg/L) of bottled sparkling or carbonated water.

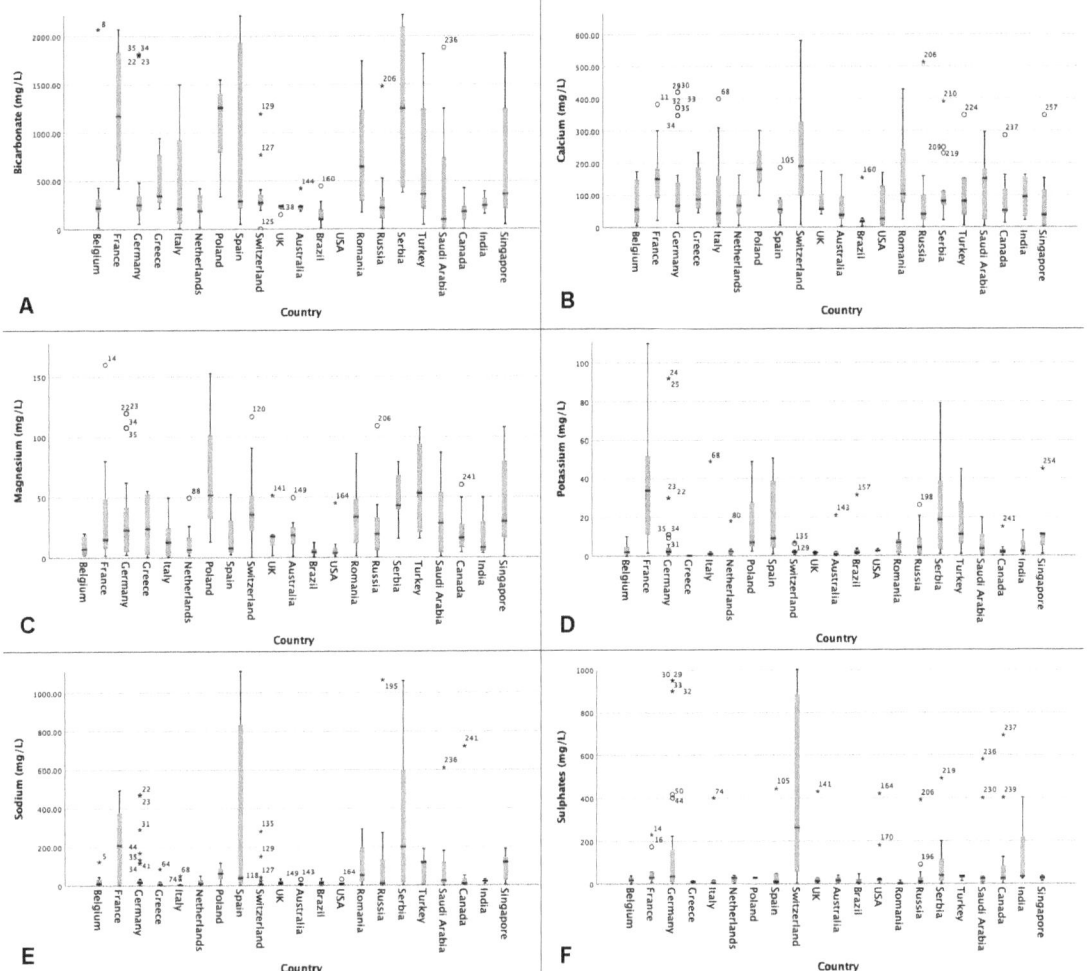

Figure 2. (A–F): The mineral composition of bottled sparkling water (mg/L) per mineral by country. ° Outlier. * Extreme value.

Overall, for sparkling or carbonated water, bicarbonate levels ranged from 0 mg/L (Aqua Mineral—Russia, 365 Days—Russia, San Pellegrino—Saudi Arabia, Voss—Saudi Arabia, Aqua—Saudi Arabia) to 7500 mg/L (Donate Mg—Serbia) worldwide. Outliers and extremes not included in Figure 2 are Borjoni (3754 mg/L), Saint Yorre (4368 mg/L) and Donat Mg (7500 mg/L).

Calcium levels ranged from 0.2 mg/L (Aqua Mineral—Russia) to 581.6 mg/L (Meltinger—Switzerland). Magnesium levels ranged from 0.2 mg/L (Zurzacher Classic—Switzerland) to 1000 mg/L (Donat Mg—Serbia). Donat Mg and Mg Miveia (343 mg/L) are excluded in Figure 2.

Potassium levels ranged from 0 mg/L (Voss—Saudi Arabia/Australia, Nestlé PureLife—Canada, Perrier—Belgium) to 195 mg/L (Ion Water—Singapore).

Sodium levels ranged from 0.3 mg/L (Montana—Saudi Arabia) to 1708 mg/L (Saint-Yorre—France). The outliers and extremes excluded in the boxplot are Donat Mg (1500 mg/L), Borjoni (1590 mg/L) and Saint Yorre (1780 mg/L).

Sulphates levels ranged from 0 mg/L (Ordal—Belgium) to 2200 mg/L (Donat Mg—Serbia). Donat Mg and Lipetsk (1320 mg/L) were the extremes excluded.

A complete overview of the mineral content of all still water brands and sparkling water brands per country, can be found in Table S1, which is submitted as Supplementary Data.

4. Discussion

This descriptive, multi-continental study conducted in 21 countries is, to our knowledge the first study to evaluate the mineral composition of commercially available bottled water worldwide. In total, 316 brands for still water and 224 brands for sparkling water were assessed. Our results show that on a global level the mineral composition of bottled drinkable water varies enormously.

On average, calcium levels of still water vary by a factor of 18.7. Considering each brand individually, a difference of 579 mg/L in calcium content was observed between brands. Moores Ultra Pure—Australia does not contain any calcium, whereas Abdelbodner Cristal—Switzerland for example contains as much as 579 mg/L. This illustrates the wide range in calcium content of commercially available bottled still water worldwide.

Calcium intake plays a significant role in bone homeostasis. A study performed by Costi et al., showed that drinking a mineral water rich in calcium (318 mg/L) significantly contributed to maintaining bone mass of the spine in postmenopausal women [27]. On the other hand, an acidic environment, which can be the result of chronic renal failure or renal tubular acidosis, provokes calcium efflux from the bone, by bone resorption leading to osteoporosis [28]. Adequate calcium intake is therefore of utmost importance for CKD patients. High calcium waters may be a calorie-free nutritional supplement for those with low calcium levels as calcium supplements were thought to increase cardiovascular (CVD) risk [29,30]. However, although the relationship between calcium intake and bone formation is clear, controversy remains whether calcium intake affects the risk for CVD as the evidence is contradictory [31–33].

The conception of calcium being a promoter of KSD has long been established. Supersaturation of the urine with calcium, or hypercalciuria, correlates directly to the formation of kidney stones, as a calcium excretion of more than 200 mg/L a day increases stone risk [17]. Consequently, urinary supersaturation of calcium results in a significant risk of recurrence [34]. Although historically a low calcium diet was advised to prevent hypercalciuria, nowadays a normal calcium intake of 1000–1200 mg/day is the standard. A lack of calcium intake through the diet results in a secondary increase in oxalate as calcium binds to oxalate in the gut. Therefore, in case of a low calcium diet, hyper-absorption of free oxalate occurs, resulting in hyperoxaluria [18,35]. A study performed by Curhan et al. showed that a low calcium diet was associated with a 34% higher risk of kidney stones [36]. As 25% of the waters included in our study contain a significant amount of calcium (>100 mg/L), it is important that KSD patients are aware of the calcium content of the water they drink.

Their calcium intake through drinking water should be included as part of the total calcium intake per day and might result in alterations of the patients' diet.

Another factor contributing to urinary calcium excretion is sodium intake. Since 1964, several studies have documented that an increase in dietary sodium is directly related to calcium excretion, especially in stone formers. An increase in sodium intake of 6 g/day, could lead to an increase in calcium excretion of 40 mg/day [37]. Furthermore, hypercalciuria was corrected in approximately 30% of idiopathic hypercalciuria patients by following a low sodium diet [38]. This phenomenon can be explained by the renal handling of sodium and calcium. Reabsorption of calcium in the distal renal tubule is dependent on sodium exchange. A high sodium load will therefore result in increased urinary calcium. Secondly, hypervolemia induced by a high sodium load might alter sodium and calcium reabsorption [37–39].

Although median sodium levels were generally low, our study did include bottled water with high sodium content. For 9 water brands, sodium levels exceeded 1000 mg/L (still water: Element—Serbia (1605 mg/L), sparkling water: Heba Strong—Serbia (1060 mg/L), Lipetsk—Russia (1065 mg/L), San Narciso—Spain (1080 mg/L), Vichy Catalan—Spain (1097 mg/L), Malavella—Spain (1115 mg/L), Donat Mg—Serbia (1500 mg/L), Borjomi—Russia (1590 mg/L), Saint-Yorre—France (1708 mg/L)). By drinking 3 L of such water, KSD patients might unintentionally increase the risk for stone formation by inducing hypercalciuria as their sodium intake, which often already exceeds the recommended daily intake, significantly increases. However, also for non-stone formers, monitoring the sodium intake is relevant as a high sodium intake of more than 5 g/day is associated with high blood pressure and significantly related to a higher risk of stroke and of end-stage kidney disease, particularly when KSD has contributed to CKD development [40].

Contrary to calcium and sodium, bicarbonate may protect against kidney stone formation. Bicarbonate as an alkaline substance increases urinary pH and stimulates citrate excretion, an inhibitor of stone formation. Earlier studies have demonstrated that consuming a mineral water rich in bicarbonate (>1715 mg/L) significantly increases urinary pH to metaphylactic levels around 6.7 [41,42]. Furthermore, the excretion of citrate, which chelates urinary calcium to form soluble complexes and also prevents aggregations of calcium oxalate, significantly increased to levels normally reached by pharmacologic treatment with sodium potassium citrate [41]. This suggests that mineral water instead of (or in combination with) pharmacologic agents could be used as a metaphylaxis therapy.

There are several water brands included in this study with such a high bicarbonate content (> 1715 mg/L), most of them being sparkling water (22 sparkling waters, three still waters). Some of these even contain extreme amounts of bicarbonate, with concentrations up to 7500 mg/L (Donat Mg—Serbia). However, a study performed by Karagülle et al. demonstrated that the ingestion of bicarbonate water with a content of 2673 mg/L also increased urinary supersaturation with calcium phosphate. Alkaline waters are not suitable for phosphate stone formers as the goal is to lower urinary pH in such patients [42].

Another mineral potentially inhibiting stone formation is magnesium. Like bicarbonate, magnesium provides for an alkali load resulting in more alkaline urine. Moreover, magnesium competes with calcium in binding to free oxalate, which increases solubility. Therefore, theoretically, magnesium can reduce oxalate reabsorption in the gut and the urinary tract to prevent precipitation of calcium oxalate [43]. However, controversy remains as several studies failed to demonstrate a decline in urinary oxalate in case of higher magnesium intake where other studies did [43].

Magnesium is a key nutrient in several biochemical processes in the body. It is involved in glucose homeostasis, lipid metabolism, neuronal functioning, bone metabolism and many more cellular processes throughout the human body [44]. Many studies have been performed to evaluate the effects of dietary magnesium on our health, including ischemic heart disease, diabetes type 2, hypertension and CKD [44]. Considering CVD risk, studies have shown that dietary magnesium is inversely related to CVD risk and fatal ischemic heart disease [16,45,46]. This also applies for patients with CKD, who are already at increased risk for cardiovascular mortality [47]. A meta-analysis performed by Gianfredi et al., evaluated the association of magnesium and calcium rich drinking water (hard water) with CVD risk. Although heterogeneity was present, the consumption of hard water could be protective regarding CVD risk [48].

Adequate potassium intake also lowers CVD risk and high potassium intake might even counterbalance for the CVD risk associated with high sodium intake. As potassium is mainly found in vegetables and fruits, this correlation might be explained by a healthy diet overall lowering cardiovascular risk [40,46].

Regarding KSD, potassium intake is inversely related to KSD risk [36]. A study performed by Ferraro et al. showed that a daily potassium intake of 2781 mg/day lowers the risk of kidney stones by 33–56% [49]. As the water currently studied did not contain as much potassium, KSD patients should predominantly rely on vegetables and fruits to achieve an adequate potassium intake.

With the increasing prevalence of KSD the management should shift more towards focusing on the prevention of recurrence. Although pharmacologic treatment with thiazide diuretics and potassium citrate is well established in the current guidelines, modification of the diet for the prevention of KSD is gaining interest [50,51]. As fluid therapy is the corner stone in the prevention of stone formation, urologists should realize that drinking water contains minerals that could affect urinary metabolites either promoting or inhibiting kidney stone formation. Furthermore, as this study shows, the mineral composition of bottled drinking water varies greatly worldwide. Therefore, effective dietary counselling on the prevention of stone recurrence should also include advice on what type of water to drink considering stone composition. Also, the differences in mineral composition between tap water versus bottled water should be addressed. Although the mineral composition of tap water does vary locally, it does not vary to such extent that it affects stone development as tap water is strictly regulated by the government. However, as shown by our study, the mineral composition of bottled water does vary enormously worldwide. Although most countries have access to tap water, the consumption of bottled water is increasing worldwide. Especially in Western countries, where good quality tap water is easily accessible, this seems paradoxical. In the US for example, the average consumption per capita has doubled to 138.17 L in 2015 [52]. In France, the consumption of bottled water per capita increased from 6 L per person in 1940 to 141 L per person in 2015, a 2350% increase [53]. Although more people are gaining access to clean tap water, a trend towards bottled water also occurs in developing countries [54].

Besides the importance of knowledge on the mineral composition of water for KSD patients to prevent stone formation, an adequate dietary mineral intake, which can be supplemented by drinking mineral water, is essential for bone health and lowering CVD risk. Although the biochemical processes in our body involving minerals like calcium, bicarbonate and magnesium are complex, maintaining a low-grade metabolic alkalosis might protect against age-related diseases as these seem to be related to acidosis [55].

To the best of our knowledge, this is the first study to analyse the mineral composition of commercially available bottled still and bottled sparkling or carbonated water worldwide. As earlier studies performed in Europe showed previously [25,26], this global study shows that the mineral composition of bottled water varies greatly worldwide. We intended to analyse the mineral content of bottled water worldwide and took samples from 21 countries. A limitation of our study is that we relied on information given by the manufacturers on the labels regarding the mineral composition of the included waters rather than independent laboratory measurements. Unfortunately, our study did not include bottled drinking water from the African continent. Also, we did not evaluate the mineral composition of tap water. It would be interesting to investigate to what extent the mineral composition of tap water differs from that of bottled drinking water globally. Secondly, it would be interesting to compare geographical differences in the mineral composition of tap water to KSD prevalence rates, CVD risk and osteoporosis worldwide. However, as there are lots of other dietary and non-dietary factors contributing to the risk of stone formation, CVD and bone health, it will be difficult to determine the exact role of the mineral composition of water on the development of disease.

5. Conclusions

KSD is a complex and multifactorial disease with increasing prevalence rates worldwide. As recurrences rates are high, the focus in management of this disease has to include strategies of prevention. Although drinking sufficient amounts of water is recommended, drinking water can contain inhibitors as well as promotors of stone formation. On the other hand, adequate dietary mineral intake is important for bone health and lowers CVD risk. As the mineral content of bottled still and bottled sparkling or carbonated water varies enormously across the globe, urologists and nephrologists should counsel their patients on an individual level regarding their water intake.

Supplementary Materials: The following are available online at https://www.mdpi.com/article/10.3390/jcm10132807/s1, Table S1: The mineral composition (mg/L) of bottled still and sparkling water by country.

Author Contributions: Conceptualization, B.K.S.; methodology, B.K.S., G.M.K. and S.J.M.S.; software, R.G.; validation, R.G., formal analysis, R.G.; investigation, R.G. and S.J.M.S.; data curation, S.J.M.S., M.M.E.L.H., B.M.Z.H., S.I., A.P. (Amelia Pietropaolo), E.J., S.M.A., S.B.H., E.V., O.T., V.G., E.X.K., V.D.C., O.D., N.K.G., L.B.D., T.E.S., N.R., M.T., P.K., E.E., E.B.-N., K.B.S., N.B., A.V., A.P. (Angela Piccirilli) and B.K.S.; writing—original draft preparation, S.J.M.S.; writing—review and editing, S.J.M.S., G.M.K., L.V and B.K.S.; supervision, G.M.K. and B.K.S.; project administration, S.J.M.S. All authors have read and agreed to the published version of the manuscript.

Funding: This research received no external funding.

Institutional Review Board Statement: Not applicable.

Informed Consent Statement: Not applicable.

Data Availability Statement: Not applicable.

Conflicts of Interest: The authors declare no conflict of interest.

References

1. Rukin, N.J.; Siddiqui, Z.A.; Chedgy, E.C.P.; Somani, B.K. Trends in Upper Tract Stone Disease in England: Evidence from the Hospital Episodes Statistics Database. *Urol. Int.* **2017**, *98*, 391–396. [CrossRef]
2. Wong, Y.; Cook, P.; Roderick, P.; Somani, B.K. Metabolic Syndrome and Kidney Stone Disease: A Systematic Review of Literature. *J. Endourol.* **2016**, *30*, 246–253. [CrossRef]
3. Sorokin, I.; Mamoulakis, C.; Miyazawa, K.; Rodgers, A.; Talati, J.; Lotan, Y. Epidemiology of stone disease across the world. *World J. Urol.* **2017**, *35*, 1301–1320. [CrossRef]
4. Ferraro, P.M.; Curhan, G.C.; D'Addessi, A.; Gambaro, G. Risk of recurrence of idiopathic calcium kidney stones: Analysis of data from the literature. *J. Nephrol.* **2017**, *30*, 227–233. [CrossRef]
5. Ferraro, P.M.; Taylor, E.N.; Eisner, B.H.; Gambaro, G.; Rimm, E.B.; Mukamal, K.J.; Curhan, G.C. History of kidney stones and the risk of coronary heart disease. *JAMA* **2013**, *310*, 408–415. [CrossRef] [PubMed]
6. Cupisti, A.; D'Alessandro, C.; Samoni, S.; Meola, M.; Egidi, M.F. Nephrolithiasis and hypertension: Possible links and clinical implications. *J. Nephrol.* **2014**, *27*, 477–482. [CrossRef]
7. Kim, S.Y.; Bang, W.J.; Min, C.; Choi, H.G. Association of nephrolithiasis with the risk of cardiovascular diseases: A longitudinal follow-up study using a national health screening cohort. *BMJ Open* **2020**, *10*, e040034. [CrossRef]
8. Sakhaee, K. Nephrolithiasis as a systemic disorder. *Curr. Opin. Nephrol. Hypertens.* **2008**, *17*, 304–309. [CrossRef]
9. Borghi, L.; Meschi, T.; Amato, F.; Briganti, A.; Novarini, A.; Giannini, A. Urinary volume, water and recurrences in idiopathic calcium nephrolithiasis: A 5-year randomized prospective study. *J. Urol.* **1996**, *155*, 839–843. [CrossRef]
10. Skolarikos, A.; Straub, M.; Knoll, T.; Sarica, K.; Seitz, C.; Petřík, A.; Türk, C. Metabolic evaluation and recurrence prevention for urinary stone patients: Eau guidelines. *Eur. Urol.* **2015**, *67*, 750–763. [CrossRef]
11. Pak, C.Y.C.; Sakhaee, K.; Crowther, C.; Brinkley, L. Evidence justifying a high fluid intake in treatment of nephrolithiasis. *Ann. Intern. Med.* **1980**, *93*, 36–39. [CrossRef]
12. Gamage, K.N.; Jamnadass, E.; Sulaiman, S.K.; Pietropaolo, A.; Aboumarzouk, O.; Somani, B.K. The role of fluid intake in the prevention of kidney stone disease: A systematic review over the last two decades. *Türk Üroloji Dergisi/Turkish J. Urol.* **2020**, *46*, S92–S103. [CrossRef]

13. Clark, W.F.; Moist, L.; Sontrop, J.M.; Huang, S.-H.; Bouby, N.; Bankir, L. Hydration and Chronic Kidney Disease Progression: A Critical Review of the Evidence. *Am. J. Nephrol.* **2016**, *43*, 281–292. [CrossRef] [PubMed]
14. Vannucci, L.; Fossi, C.; Quattrini, S.; Guasti, L.; Pampaloni, B.; Gronchi, G.; Giusti, F.; Romagnoli, C.; Cianferotti, L.; Marcucci, G.; et al. Calcium Intake in Bone Health: A Focus on Calcium-Rich Mineral Waters. *Nutrients* **2018**, *10*, 1930. [CrossRef] [PubMed]
15. Wynn, E.; Krieg, M.-A.; Aeschlimann, J.-M.; Burckhardt, P. Alkaline mineral water lowers bone resorption even in calcium sufficiency. *Bone* **2009**, *44*, 120–124. [CrossRef]
16. Jiang, L.; He, P.; Chen, J.; Liu, Y.; Liu, D.; Qin, G.; Tan, N. Magnesium Levels in Drinking Water and Coronary Heart Disease Mortality Risk: A Meta-Analysis. *Nutrients* **2016**, *8*, 5. [CrossRef]
17. Coe, F.L.; Worcester, F.L.C.E.M.; Evan, A.P. Idiopathic hypercalciuria and formation of calcium renal stones. *Nat. Rev. Nephrol.* **2016**, *12*, 519–533. [CrossRef]
18. Ferraro, P.M.; Bargagli, M.; Trinchieri, A.; Gambaro, G. Risk of Kidney Stones: Influence of Dietary Factors, Dietary Patterns, and Vegetarian–Vegan Diets. *Nutrients* **2020**, *12*, 779. [CrossRef]
19. Prezioso, D.; Strazzullo, P.; Lotti, T.; Bianchi, G.; Borghi, L.; Caione, P.; Carini, M.; Caudarella, R.; Gambaro, G.; Gelosa, M.; et al. Dietary treatment of urinary risk factors for renal stone formation. A review of CLU Working Group. *Arch. Ital. Urol. Androl.* **2015**, *87*, 105–120. [CrossRef]
20. Goldfarb, D.S. Empiric therapy for kidney stones. *Urolithiasis* **2019**, *47*, 107–113. [CrossRef]
21. Ferraro, P.M.; Taylor, E.N.; Gambaro, G.; Curhan, G.C. Soda and Other Beverages and the Risk of Kidney Stones. *Clin. J. Am. Soc. Nephrol. CJASN* **2013**, *8*, 1389–1395. [CrossRef]
22. Rodríguez, F.M.; Garcia, S.G.; Corro, R.J.; Liesa, M.S.; Barón, F.R.; Martín, F.S.; Feu, O.A.; Rodríguez, R.M.; Mavrich, H.V. Análisis de las aguas embotelladas y de grifo españolas y de las implicaciones de su consumo en la litiasis urinaria. *Actas Urol. Esp.* **2009**, *33*, 778–793. [CrossRef]
23. Hubert, J. Drinking water: Which type should be chosen? *Prog. Urol.* **2010**, *20*, 806–809. [CrossRef]
24. Azoulay, A.; Garzon, P.; Eisenberg, M.J. Comparison of the mineral content of tap water and bottled waters. *J. Gen. Intern. Med.* **2001**, *16*, 168–175. [CrossRef]
25. Stoots, S.J.; Geraghty, R.; Kamphuis, G.M.; Jamnadass, E.; Henderickx, M.M.; Ventimiglia, E.; Traxer, O.; Keller, E.X.; De Coninck, V.; Talso, M.; et al. Variations in the Mineral Content of Bottled "Still" Water Across Europe: Comparison of 182 Brands Across 10 Countries. *J. Endourol.* **2021**, *35*, 206–214. [CrossRef]
26. Stoots, S.J.; Geraghty, R.; Kamphuis, G.M.; Jamnadass, E.; Henderickx, M.M.; Ventimiglia, E.; Traxer, O.; Keller, E.X.; De Coninck, V.; Talso, M.; et al. Variations in the mineral content of bottled 'carbonated or sparkling' water across Europe: A comparison of 126 brands across 10 countries. *Cent. Eur. J. Urol.* **2021**, *74*, 71–75. [CrossRef]
27. Costi, D.; Calcaterra, P.G.; Iori, N.; Vourna, S.; Nappi, G.; Passeri, M. Importance of bioavailable calcium drinking water for the maintenance of bone mass in post-menopausal women. *J. Endocrinol. Investig.* **1999**, *22*, 852–856. [CrossRef]
28. Bushinsky, D.A.; Frick, K.K. The effects of acid on bone. *Curr. Opin. Nephrol. Hypertens.* **2000**, *9*, 369–379. [CrossRef]
29. Xiao, Q.; Murphy, R.A.; Houston, D.; Harris, T.B.; Chow, W.-H.; Park, Y. Dietary and supplemental calcium intake and cardiovascular disease mortality. *JAMA Intern. Med.* **2013**, *173*, 639–646. [CrossRef]
30. Michaëlsson, K.; Melhus, H.; Lemming, E.W.; Wolk, A.; Byberg, L. Long term calcium intake and rates of all cause and cardiovascular mortality: Community based prospective longitudinal cohort study. *BMJ* **2013**, *346*, f228. [CrossRef]
31. Chung, M.; Tang, A.M.; Fu, Z.; Wang, D.D.; Newberry, S.J. Calcium Intake and Cardiovascular Disease Risk. *Ann. Intern. Med.* **2016**, *165*, 856–866. [CrossRef]
32. Myung, S.-K.; Kim, H.-B.; Lee, Y.-J.; Choi, Y.-J.; Oh, S.-W. Calcium Supplements and Risk of Cardiovascular Disease: A Meta-Analysis of Clinical Trials. *Nutrients* **2021**, *13*, 368. [CrossRef] [PubMed]
33. Yang, C.; Shi, X.; Xia, H.; Yang, X.; Liu, H.; Pan, D.; Sun, G. The Evidence and Controversy Between Dietary Calcium Intake and Calcium Supplementation and the Risk of Cardiovascular Disease: A Systematic Review and Meta-Analysis of Cohort Studies and Randomized Controlled Trials. *J. Am. Coll. Nutr.* **2019**, *39*, 352–370. [CrossRef]
34. Ferraro, P.M.; Ticinesi, A.; Meschi, T.; Rodgers, A.; Di Maio, F.; Fulignati, P.; Borghi, L.; Gambaro, G. Short-Term Changes in Urinary Relative Supersaturation Predict Recurrence of Kidney Stones: A Tool to Guide Preventive Measures in Urolithiasis. *J. Urol.* **2018**, *200*, 1082–1087. [CrossRef]
35. Borghi, L.; Schianchi, T.; Meschi, T.; Guerra, A.; Allegri, F.; Maggiore, U.; Novarini, A. Comparison of Two Diets for the Prevention of Recurrent Stones in Idiopathic Hypercalciuria. *N. Engl. J. Med.* **2002**, *346*, 77–84. [CrossRef]
36. Curhan, G.C.; Willett, W.C.; Rimm, E.B.; Stampfer, M.J. A Prospective Study of Dietary Calcium and Other Nutrients and the Risk of Symptomatic Kidney Stones. *N. Engl. J. Med.* **1993**, *328*, 833–838. [CrossRef]
37. Ticinesi, A.; Nouvenne, A.; Maalouf, N.M.; Borghi, L.; Meschi, T. Salt and nephrolithiasis. *Nephrol. Dial. Transplant.* **2016**, *31*, 39–45. [CrossRef]
38. Nouvenne, A.; Meschi, T.; Prati, B.; Guerra, A.; Allegri, F.; Vezzoli, G.; Soldati, L.; Gambaro, G.; Maggiore, U.; Borghi, L. Effects of a low-salt diet on idiopathic hypercalciuria in calcium-oxalate stone formers: A 3-mo randomized controlled trial. *Am. J. Clin. Nutr.* **2009**, *91*, 565–570. [CrossRef]
39. Bonny, O.; Edwards, A. Calcium reabsorption in the distal tubule: Regulation by sodium, pH, and flow. *Am. J. Physiol. Physiol.* **2013**, *304*, F585–F600. [CrossRef]

40. Mente, A.; O'Donnell, M.; Rangarajan, S.; McQueen, M.; Dagenais, G.; Wielgosz, A.; Lear, S.; Ah, S.T.L.; Wei, L.; Diaz, R.; et al. Urinary sodium excretion, blood pressure, cardiovascular disease, and mortality: A community-level prospective epidemiological cohort study. *Lancet* **2018**, *392*, 496–506. [CrossRef]
41. Keßler, T.; Hesse, A. Cross-over study of the influence of bicarbonate-rich mineral water on urinary composition in comparison with sodium potassium citrate in healthy male subjects. *Br. J. Nutr.* **2000**, *84*, 865–871. [CrossRef]
42. Karagülle, O.; Smorag, U.; Candir, F.; Gundermann, G.; Jonas, U.; Becker, A.J.; Gehrke, A.; Gutenbrunner, C. Clinical study on the effect of mineral waters containing bicarbonate on the risk of urinary stone formation in patients with multiple episodes of CaOx-urolithiasis. *World J. Urol.* **2007**, *25*, 315–323. [CrossRef] [PubMed]
43. Tavasoli, S.; Taheri, M.; Taheri, F.; Basiri, A.; Amiri, F.B. Evaluating the associations between urinary excretion of magnesium and that of other components in calcium stone-forming patients. *Int. Urol. Nephrol.* **2018**, *51*, 279–284. [CrossRef]
44. Glasdam, S.-M.; Glasdam, S.; Peters, G.H. The Importance of Magnesium in the Human Body. *Adv. Virus Res.* **2016**, *73*, 169–193. [CrossRef]
45. Del Gobbo, L.C.; Imamura, F.; Wu, J.H.Y.; Otto, M.C.D.O.; E Chiuve, S.; Mozaffarian, D. Circulating and dietary magnesium and risk of cardiovascular disease: A systematic review and meta-analysis of prospective studies. *Am. J. Clin. Nutr.* **2013**, *98*, 160–173. [CrossRef]
46. Pickering, R.; Bradlee, M.; Singer, M.; Moore, L. Higher Intakes of Potassium and Magnesium, but Not Lower Sodium, Reduce Cardiovascular Risk in the Framingham Offspring Study. *Nutrients* **2021**, *13*, 269. [CrossRef] [PubMed]
47. Leenders, N.H.; Vermeulen, E.A.; van Ballegooijen, A.J.; Hoekstra, T.; de Vries, R.; Beulens, J.W.; Vervloet, M.G. The association between circulating magnesium and clinically relevant outcomes in patients with chronic kidney disease: A systematic review and meta-analysis. *Clin. Nutr.* **2021**, *40*, 3133–3147. [CrossRef]
48. Gianfredi, V.; Bragazzi, N.L.; Nucci, D.; Villarini, M.; Moretti, M. Cardiovascular diseases and hard drinking waters: Implications from a systematic review with meta-analysis of case-control studies. *J. Water Health* **2016**, *15*, 31–40. [CrossRef]
49. Ferraro, P.M.; Mandel, E.I.; Curhan, G.C.; Gambaro, G.; Taylor, E.N. Dietary Protein and Potassium, Diet–Dependent Net Acid Load, and Risk of Incident Kidney Stones. *Clin. J. Am. Soc. Nephrol.* **2016**, *11*, 1834–1844. [CrossRef]
50. Pearle, M.S.; Goldfarb, D.; Assimos, D.G.; Curhan, G.; Denu-Ciocca, C.J.; Matlaga, B.R.; Monga, M.; Penniston, K.L.; Preminger, G.M.; Turk, T.M.; et al. Medical Management of Kidney Stones: AUA Guideline. *J. Urol.* **2014**, *192*, 316–324. [CrossRef]
51. Türk, C.; Neisius, A.; Petřík, A.; Seitz, C.; Thomas, K.; Skolarikos, A. EAU Guidelines on Urolithiasis 2020. In *European Association of Urology Guidelines*, 2020th ed.; vol presented at the EAU Annual Congress Amsterdam 2020; The European Association of Urology Guidelines Office: Arnhem, The Netherlands, 2020.
52. Qian, N. Bottled Water or Tap Water? A Comparative Study of Drinking Water Choices on University Campuses. *Water* **2018**, *10*, 59. [CrossRef]
53. Brei, V.A. How is a bottled water market created? *WIREs Water* **2018**, *5*, e1220. [CrossRef]
54. Arnold, E.; Larsen, J. Bottled Water: Pouring Resources down the Drain. 2006. Available online: http://www.earth-policy.org/plan_b_updates/2006/update51/a/p (accessed on 20 May 2021).
55. Frassetto, L.; Morris, R.C., Jr.; Sellmeyer, D.E.; Todd, K.; Sebastian, A. Diet, evolution and aging–the pathophysiologic effects of the post-agricultural inversion of the potassium-to-sodium and base-to-chloride ratios in the human diet. *Eur. J. Nutr.* **2001**, *40*, 200–213. [CrossRef] [PubMed]

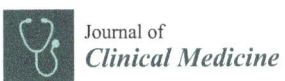

Article

Outcomes of Ureteroscopy and Laser Stone Fragmentation (URSL) for Kidney Stone Disease (KSD): Comparative Cohort Study Using MOSES Technology 60 W Laser System versus Regular Holmium 20 W Laser

Amelia Pietropaolo, Thomas Hughes, Mriganka Mani and Bhaskar Somani *

Department of Urology, University Hospital Southampton, Southampton SO16 6YD, UK; ameliapietr@gmail.com (A.P.); t.hughes@doctors.org.uk (T.H.); mrigankamani@gmail.com (M.M.)
* Correspondence: bhaskar.somani@uhs.nhs.uk or b.k.somani@soton.ac.uk

Abstract: Background: For ureteroscopy and laser stone fragmentation (URSL), the use of laser technology has shifted from low power to higher power lasers and the addition of Moses technology, that allows for 'fragmentation, dusting and pop-dusting' of stones. We wanted to compare the outcomes of URSL for Moses technology 60 W laser system versus matched regular Holmium 20 W laser cases. Methods: Prospective data were collected for patients who underwent URSL using a Moses 60 W laser (Group A) and matched to historical control data using a regular Holmium 20 W laser (Group B), performed by a single surgeon. Data were collected for patient demographics, stone location, size, pre- and post-operative stent, operative time, length of stay, complications and stone free rate (SFR). Results: A total of 38 patients in each group underwent the URSL procedure. The stones were matched for their location (17 renal and 11 ureteric stones). The mean single and cumulative stone sizes (mm) were 10.9 ± 4.4 and 15.5 ± 9.9, and 11.8 ± 4.0 and 16.5 ± 11.3 for groups A and B, respectively. The mean operative time (min) was 51.6 ± 17.1 and 82.1 ± 27.0 ($p \leq 0.0001$) for groups A and B. The initial SFR was 97.3% and 81.6% for groups A and B, respectively ($p = 0.05$), with 1 and 7 patients in each group needing a second procedure ($p = 0.05$), for a final SFR of 100% and 97.3%. While there were 2 and 5 Clavien I/II complications for groups A and B, none of the patients in group A had any infection related complication. Conclusions: Use of Moses technology with higher power was significantly faster for stone lithotripsy and reduced operative time and the number of patients who needed a second procedure to achieve a stone free status. It seems that the use of Moses technology with a mid-power laser is likely to set a new benchmark for treating complex stones, without the need for secondary procedures in most patients.

Keywords: kidney calculi; ureteroscopy; laser; RIRS; Moses; holmium

Citation: Pietropaolo, A.; Hughes, T.; Mani, M.; Somani, B. Outcomes of Ureteroscopy and Laser Stone Fragmentation (URSL) for Kidney Stone Disease (KSD): Comparative Cohort Study Using MOSES Technology 60 W Laser System versus Regular Holmium 20 W Laser. *J. Clin. Med.* **2021**, *10*, 2742. https://doi.org/10.3390/jcm10132742

Academic Editor: Emilio Sacco

Received: 27 May 2021
Accepted: 15 June 2021
Published: 22 June 2021

Publisher's Note: MDPI stays neutral with regard to jurisdictional claims in published maps and institutional affiliations.

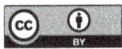

Copyright: © 2021 by the authors. Licensee MDPI, Basel, Switzerland. This article is an open access article distributed under the terms and conditions of the Creative Commons Attribution (CC BY) license (https://creativecommons.org/licenses/by/4.0/).

1. Introduction

The prevalence of kidney stone disease (KSD) has increased worldwide with a lifetime risk in Europe of up to 14% [1]. Ureteroscopy and laser stone fragmentation (URSL) has also seen a big rise over the last two decades [2]. This is attributed partly to the wide availability of holmium:YAG (Ho:YAG) laser systems since its introduction for laser lithotripsy in 1992 [3]. URSL is the first line treatment for large ureteric stones and renal stones up to 2 cm [4,5]. Compared to low power laser lithotripsy, high power lasers seem to require shorter operative time for similar outcomes [6]. The modern high powered Ho:YAG lasers can be equipped with Moses technology, which divides the laser pulse into two peaks. The first pulse separates the fluid in front of the stone (Moses effect), and the second pulse is delivered directly to the stone unimpeded by the intervening fluid, leading to better fragmentation, lower retropulsion and less time taken for the procedure [7–9].

Previous in vitro work with Moses technology has shown it to deliver increased stone ablation in soft stones when in contact and 1 mm from the stone [9]. Another in vitro study showed Moses mode to reduce stone movement by 50 times at 0.8 J and 10 Hz, which was seen in both fragmentation and dusting settings [10]. They carried out their work in porcine kidneys to show less ureteral damage on histological analysis after direct lasering of soft tissue, thereby offering safer lithotripsy in shorter time.

The use of laser technique has also evolved and includes dusting, popcorning and pop-dusting [11,12]. The use of laser technology has also shifted from low power to higher power lasers and the addition of Moses technology, which allows for 'fragmentation, dusting and pop-dusting' of stones [12]. With high power laser, higher frequency and long pulse allow for the latter, a technique which is now used for large stone treatment in a single setting [12]. A recent systematic review showed that, while high power lasers were faster, this advantage was lost for larger stones [6]. We wanted to compare the outcomes of URSL for Moses technology 60 W laser system versus matched regular Holmium 20 W laser cases. Our hypothesis was that the Moses 60 W laser would achieve better outcomes than the smaller 20 W laser system.

2. Methods

Our ureteroscopy outcome audit was registered with 'Clinical Effectiveness and Audit' department of our hospital and patient consent was taken for this purpose. Patient outcomes were collected prospectively and recorded in our database, which was then analyzed retrospectively for patient demographics, stone parameters, pre-operative assessment, operative details, laser system used, stone-free rate (SFR), length of stay (LoS), and complication rates.

Patients underwent URSL for ureteral and renal stones using a Moses 60 W laser (Group A) matched to historical control data using a regular Holmium 20 W laser (Group B), performed by a single surgeon (BS) and analysed by a third party (TH) not involved in the original procedure. Patients in Groups A and B had their procedure between March 2012 and May 2014, and August 2019 and October 2020, respectively. LoS was defined from completion of URS to their discharge, with 'day case' defined as patients who went home the same day as their surgery [13]. Data were recorded in a Microsoft Excel 2016 (Microsoft, Redmond, WA, USA) and analysed using SPSS version 26 (IBM, Armonk, NY, USA). The independent t-test, Mann–Whitney-U test, Chi-squared, and Fisher's exact test were used with a p-value of <0.05 considered statistically significant.

2.1. Pre-Operative Assessment

The diagnosis of stone was made on non-contrast CT (CTKUB) for adults and ultrasound (USS) for paediatric patients (<16 years). Positive pre-operative urine culture was treated appropriately based on the sensitivity analysis. All patients also had pre-assessment in dedicated anaesthetic led clinics.

2.2. Surgical Technique

A pre-surgical brief was done on the day as per the World Health Organisation (WHO) checklist with the theatre and recovery team where a clear plan was made regarding antibiotic prophylaxis, venous thromboembolism (VTE) prophylaxis and any anticipated surgical or anaesthetic issues.

A protocol-based procedure was done for all patients under general anaesthetic. After initial cystoscopy and safety wire placement, a rigid URS was done using 4.5 or 6F Wolf or Storz semi-rigid ureteroscope over a working wire. For renal stones, based on surgeon discretion, a ureteral access sheath (UAS) was used (9.5F/11.5F or 12F/14F Cook Flexor sheath). A flexible ureteroscopy (Storz FlexX2) and laser (Lumenis, Ltd. Yokneam, Hakidma, Israel) stone treatment was then done using a Moses P60W laser (Group A) or Holmium 20 W laser (Group B). The laser setting used was 0.4–0.8 J, 20–35 Hz with Moses setting for group A and 0.4–0.8 J, 12–18 Hz for group B. Fragments were retrieved using Cook Ngage stone extractor (Cook Medical, Bloomington, IN, USA), with a 6F ureteral stent placed post-operatively when indicated.

2.3. Post-Procedural Outcomes

SFR was defined as complete clearance of stones endoscopically and ≤2 mm fragments on post-operative imaging done 2–4 months later. While radiopaque stones were followed up with a plain radiograph, radiolucent stone follow-up was done using an ultrasound scan. If ambiguity remained and patients had symptoms, a CT scan was then done. All intra and post-operative complications were recorded, the latter classified as per the Clavien–Dindo classification system.

3. Results

A total of 76 patients (38 patients in each group) underwent a URSL procedure (Table 1). The stones were matched for their location with 17 renal and 11 ureteric stones in each group. The mean age for groups A and B were 53.8 ± 5.8 and 58.1 ± 14.5 years, respectively, with a male:female ratio of 21:17 and 25:13 in the two groups.

The mean single and cumulative stone sizes (mm) were 10.9 ± 4.4 and 15.5 ± 9.9, and 11.8 ± 4.0 and 16.5 ± 11.3 for groups A and B, respectively, with 10 and 9 patients having multiple stones. The pre and post-operative stent rates were 26.3% and 34.2%, and 86.8% and 97.3% for groups A and B, respectively. The mean operative time (min) was 51.6 ± 17.1 and 82.1 ± 27.0 ($p \leq 0.0001$) for groups A and B. The SFR was 97.3% and 81.6% for groups A and B, respectively ($p = 0.05$), with 1 and 7 patients in each group needing a second procedure ($p = 0.05$), for a final SFR of 100% and 97.3% in both the groups. While there were 2 (5.2%) and 5 (13.1%) complications for groups A and B, none of the patients in group A had any infection related complication. The complications in group A related to stent pain ($n = 2$), and group B related to urosepsis ($n = 2$), urinary tract infection ($n = 2$) and pyelonephritis ($n = 1$).

Table 1. Patient and procedural details (PUJ—pelviureteric junction, LP—lower pole, MP—mid pole, LP—lower pole, UA—uric acid, COM—Calcium oxalate monohydrate, COD—calcium oxalate dihydrate, CPC—calcium phosphate carbonate, CHP—calcium hydrogen phosphate dihydrate, MAH—magnesium ammonium phosphate).

	MOSES 60 W (Group A)	Holmium 20 W (Group B)	
Number	38	38	
Age mean ± SD (range), years	53.8 ± 5.8, (9–81)	58.1 ± 14.5, (22–84)	$p = 0.26$
Gender: Male:Female	21 (55.3%): 17 (44.7%)	25 (65.7%): 13 (34.3%)	$p = 0.35$
Side: Left: Right: Bilateral	21:16:1	22:15:1	$p = 0.97$
Location Ureter PUJ:LP:MP:UP Multiple	11 4:8:3:2 10	11 9:4:4:1 9	$p = 0.52$
Single stone size (mm) Mean ±SD (range)	10.9 ± 4.4 (4–24)	11.8 ± 4.0 (4–20)	$p = 0.34$
Cumulative stone length (mm) Mean ±SD (range)	15.5 ± 9.9 (4–57)	16.5 ± 11.3 (5–58)	$p = 0.63$
Number of stones mean ±SD (range)	2.0 ± 2.0 (1–11)	1.8 ± 1.3 (1–7)	$p = 0.51$
Pre-op stent	10 (26.3%)	13 (34.2%)	$p = 0.45$
Post-op stent	33 (86.8%)	37 (97.3%)	$p = 0.20$
Ureteral access sheath	22 (57.8%)	21 (55.2%)	$p = 0.82$
Operation time (min) mean± SD (range)	51.6 ± 17.1 (16–90)	82.1 ± 27.0 (40–160)	$p \leq 0.0001$

Table 1. Cont.

	MOSES 60 W (Group A)	Holmium 20 W (Group B)	
Initial Stone Free rate (SFR)	37 (97.3%)	31 (81.6%)	$p = 0.05$
Final SFR	38 (100%)	37 (97.3%)	
Patients requiring 2nd procedure	1 (2.6%)	7 (18.4%)	$p = 0.05$
Length of stay (LOS) (days) median (range)	0 (0–2)	0 (0–6)	$p = 0.26$
Stone analysis			
UA + COM	3	1	
COM	15	7	
COD + COM + CPC	1	1	
COD + CHP + COM	2	1	
COD + CPC	3	1	
COM + COD	2	3	
COM + CPC	8	9	
CPC + MAH	1	6	
Cystine	2	2	
UA	0	1	
Complications (%)	2 (5.2%)	5 (13.1%)	$p = 0.43$
Pain	2	0	Clavien I
Urosepsis	0	2	Clavien II
UTI	0	2	Clavien II
Pyelonephritis	0	1	Clavien II

4. Discussion

4.1. Meaning of the Study

This study is one of the first to use 60 W Moses Ho:YAG laser in the clinical setting. When compared to the 20 W laser, it was 57% faster (51.6 min versus 82.1 min, $p < 0.0001$) for comparable mean cumulative stone sizes of over 15 mm for both groups. A second procedure was needed for 1 and 7 patients, respectively, for groups A and B ($p = 0.05$) for achieving a SFR of 100% and 97.3%, suggesting a better first-time stone clearance with the 60 W Moses laser. Although not statistically significant, none of the patients in group A had infection related complication compared to 5 in group B. The latter group also had a slightly higher rate of pre- and post-operative stent usage.

4.2. Role of Moses Technology and High-Power Laser

Recently, a number of studies have shown the advantage of using both Moses technology and high-power laser for stone fragmentation (6,7,12). With the use of dusting and pop-dusting techniques, large stones (≥ 15 mm) were treated with a mean operative time of 51 min and an initial SFR of 93% [12]. Using a 120 W generator with 200 micron fiber, a randomised clinical trial (RCT) compared Moses versus regular mode laser lithotripsy for 72 patients. While the total energy and lasing times were similar, Moses mode was associated with significantly less retropulsion ($p = 0.01$), fragmentation/pulverization time ($p = 0.03$) and procedural time ($p = 0.03$) [7]. A recent study comparing 120 W laser with and without Moses mode for benign prostate hyperplasia (BPH) showed better haemostasis and same day discharge with the former [14].

4.3. Emerging Advancements in Laser Techniques and Technology

From the early stages of low powered laser lithotripsy, there is now increasing reliance on high power lasers with pulse modulation and newer techniques of fragmentation [15]. The Moses technology has been shown to increase fragmentation and reduce retropulsion. There is now emergence of a thulium fiber laser (TFL) which allows improvements in ablation efficiency and retropulsion with the added advantage of portability, and while more clinical studies need to be done, it has increased the playing field of the laser market giving more choice to the endourologists [16]. Recently, a study from Russia showed the efficacy of TFL for ureteral stones with the authors recommending a setting of 0.5 J, 30 Hz for fragmentation and 0.15 J and 100 Hz for dusting [17]. Another study for TFL on 50 patients showed the safety and efficacy for both ureteral and renal stones [18].

4.4. Strengths, Limitations and Areas of Future Research

While this study comes from a single centre and surgeon, it is limited by the retrospective nature of the study design. Apart from the laser, all equipment, techniques and armamentarium used were exactly the same in both time periods. All patients followed the same pathway with their pre-operative assessment and post-operative care. A higher incidence of post-operative infectious complications could be partly explained by higher procedural duration in group B, which is a known pre-disposing factor for this [19]. Similarly, although not significant, group B also had patients with slightly larger stones and higher proportion of patients with pre- and post-operative stents and struvite stones, which are all risk factors for infectious complications [20,21]. Nevertheless, there was a higher SFR and lower secondary procedure rates in group B, suggesting the procedural advantage offered by the 60 W Moses technology when compared to the 20 W technology. In a previous study, procedural time saving did not result in an overall cost saving, which was offset by the cost of the Moses technology [22]. However, this study did not factor the cost associated with the need for secondary procedures. The significantly shorter operative time may increase capacity on operating lists, thereby reducing the time patients are required to wait for their operation, which is beneficial to patients given the substantial impact KSD can have on quality of life [23].

Future studies should ideally be designed as an RCT and consider other aspects such as cost and quality of life, with an emphasis on standardising the outcome measure such as SFR and imaging used to achieve it. Ideally, the SFR should be assessed by a CT scan rather than XR or ultrasound scan. While the role of high-power laser in the field of BPH is more defined, it remains uncertain on the level of advantage it gives to stone surgery. Perhaps a more defined cost-analysis on the cost of machine, laser fiber, scope purchase and repair costs, the cost of procedural time and need for secondary procedure would determine the true value offered by the high-power laser and Moses technology [24,25]. Until then, the 60 W Moses laser might offer a trade-off between cost incurred and outcomes achieved for stone procedures.

5. Conclusions

The use of Moses technology with higher power was significantly faster for stone lithotripsy and reduced operative time and the number of patients who needed a second procedure to achieve a stone free status. It seems that the use of Moses technology with a mid-power laser is likely to set a new benchmark for treating large stones, bilateral or multiple stones in a single setting, without the need for secondary procedures in most patients. The exact role of different laser technologies and techniques must be defined for ease of understanding and use in clinical practice.

Author Contributions: Conseptulization—A.P., B.S.; Methodology—T.H., A.P.; Formal Analysis—T.H.; Review and editing—A.P., T.H., M.M., B.S.; Supervision—B.S. All authors have read and agreed to the published version of the manuscript.

Funding: This research received no funding.

Institutional Review Board Statement: Our study was registered as an audit with the hospital audit and clinical effectiveness department.

Informed Consent Statement: All patients were consented for their participation in any possible audit or research projects.

Data Availability Statement: Data is available and kept in the hospital electronic system.

Conflicts of Interest: Educational grant for the paper was received by AP and BS. No funding was received for the conduct of this project. The laser machine was given to the urology department for the conduct of the study.

References

1. Rukin, N.J.; Siddiqui, Z.A.; Chedgy, E.C.; Somani, B.K. Trends in Upper Tract Stone Disease in England: Evidence from the Hospital Episodes Statistics (HES) Database. *Urol. Int.* **2017**, *98*, 391–396. [CrossRef]
2. Geraghty, R.; Jones, P.; Somani, B.K. Worldwide Trends of Urinary Stone Disease Treatment over the last two Decades: A Sys-tematic Review. *J. Endourol.* **2017**, *31*, 547–556. [CrossRef]
3. Johnson, D.E.; Cromeens, D.M.; Price, R.E. Use of the holmium:YAG laser in urology. *Lasers Surg. Med.* **1992**, *12*, 353–363. [CrossRef]
4. Turk, C.; Neisius, A.; Petrik, A.; Sarica, K.; Skolarikos, A.; Straub, M.; Seitz, C. EAU Guidelines on Urolithiasis. Available online: https://uroweb.org/wp-content/uploads/EAU-Guidelines-on-Urolithiasis-2021.pdf (accessed on 15 June 2021).
5. Assimos, D.; Krambeck, A.; Miller, N.L.; Monga, M.; Murad, M.H.; Nelson, C.P.; Pace, K.T.; Pais, V.M., Jr.; Pearle, M.S.; Preminger, G.M.; et al. Surgical Management of Stones: AUA/Endourology Society Guideline. Available online: https://www.auanet.org/guidelines/kidney-stones-surgical-management-guideline (accessed on 15 June 2021).
6. Ventimiglia, E.; Pauchard, F.; Quadrini, F.; Sindhubodee, S.; Kamkoum, H.; Godínez, A.J.; Doizi, S.; Traxer, O. High- and Low-Power Laser Lithotripsy Achieves Similar Results: A Systematic Review and Meta-Analysis of Available Clinical Series. *J. Endourol.* **2021**. [CrossRef]
7. Ibrahim, A.; Badaan, S.; Elhilali, M.M.; Andonian, S. Moses technology in a stone simulator. *Can. Urol. Assoc. J.* **2017**, *12*, 127–130. [CrossRef]
8. Keller, E.X.; De Coninck, V.; Audouin, M.; Doizi, S.; Bazin, D.; Daudon, M.; Traxer, O. Fragments and dust after Holmium laser lithotripsy with or without "Moses technology": How are they different? *J. Biophotonics* **2018**, *12*, e201800227. [CrossRef]
9. Winship, B.; Wollin, D.A.; Carlos, E.C.; Li, J.; Peters, C.; Simmons, W.N.; Preminger, G.M.; Lipkin, M.E. Dusting Efficiency of the Moses Holmium Laser: An Automated In Vitro Assessment. *J. Endourol.* **2018**, *32*, 1131–1135. [CrossRef]
10. Elhilali, M.M.; Badaan, S.; Ibrahim, A.; Andonian, S. Use of the Moses Technology to Improve Holmium Laser Lithotripsy Outcomes: A Preclinical Study. *J. Endourol.* **2017**, *31*, 598–604. [CrossRef]
11. Kronenberg, P.; Somani, B. Advances in Lasers for the Treatment of Stones—a Systematic Review. *Curr. Urol. Rep.* **2018**, *19*, 1–11. [CrossRef]
12. Pietropaolo, A.; Jones, P.; Whitehurst, L.; Somani, B.K. Role of 'Dusting and Pop-Dusting' using a high powered (100W) laser machine in the treatment of large stones (≥15mm): Prospective outcomes over 16-months. *Urolithiasis* **2019**, *47*, 391–394. [CrossRef]
13. Ghosh, A.; Oliver, R.; Way, C.; White, L.; Somani, B.K. Results of day-case ureterorenoscopy (DC-URS) for stone disease: Prospective outcomes over 4.5 years. *World J. Urol.* **2017**, *35*, 1757–1764. [CrossRef]
14. Nottingham, C.U.; Large, T.; Agarwal, D.K.; Rivera, M.E.; Krambeck, A. Comparison of Newly-Optimized Moses Technology Versus Standard Holmium: YAG for Endoscopic Laser Enucleation of the Prostate. *J. Endourol.* **2021**. [CrossRef]
15. Aldoukhi, A.H.; Black, K.M.; Ghani, K.R. Emerging Laser Techniques for the Management of Stones. *Urol. Clin. N. Am.* **2019**, *46*, 193–205. [CrossRef]
16. Kronenberg, P.; Hameed, B.Z.; Somani, B. Outcomes of thulium fibre laser for treatment of urinary tract stones: Results of a systematic review. *Curr. Opin. Urol.* **2021**, *31*, 80–86. [CrossRef]
17. Enikeev, D.; Grigoryan, V.; Fokin, I.; Morozov, A.; Taratkin, M.; Klimov, R.; Kozlov, V.; Gabdullina, S.; Glybochko, P. Endoscopic lithotripsy with a superpulsed thulium fiber laser for ureteral stones: A single-centre experience. *Int. J. Urol.* **2021**, *28*, 261–265. [CrossRef] [PubMed]
18. Corrales, M.; Traxer, O. Initial clinical experience with the new thulium fiber laser: First 50 cases. *World J. Urol.* **2021**, 1–6. [CrossRef]
19. Chugh, S.; Pietropaolo, A.; Montanari, E.; Sarica, K.; Somani, B.K. Predictors of Urinary Infections and Urosepsis After Ureteroscopy for Stone Disease: A Systematic Review from EAU Section of Urolithiasis (EULIS). *Curr. Urol. Rep.* **2020**, *21*, 16–18. [CrossRef]
20. Nevo, A.; Mano, R.; Baniel, J.; Lifshitz, D.A. Ureteric stent dwelling time: A risk factor for post-ureteroscopy sepsis. *BJU Int.* **2017**, *120*, 117–122. [CrossRef] [PubMed]
21. De Coninck, V.; Keller, E.X.; Somani, B.; Giusti, G.; Proietti, S.; Rodriguez-Socarras, M.; Rodríguez-Monsalve, M.; Doizi, S.; Ventimiglia, E.; Traxer, O. Complications in Ureteroscopy: A complete overview. *World J. Urol.* **2020**, *38*, 2147–2166. [CrossRef]
22. Stern, K.L.; Monga, M. The Moses holmium system—time is money. *Can. J. Urol.* **2018**, *25*, 9313–9316.
23. New, F.; Somani, B.K. A Complete World Literature Review of Quality of Life (QoL) in Patients with Kidney Stone Disease (KSD). *Curr. Urol. Rep.* **2016**, *17*, 88. [CrossRef] [PubMed]
24. Somani, B.K.; Robertson, A.; Kata, S.G. Decreasing the Cost of Flexible Ureterorenoscopic Procedures. *Urology* **2011**, *78*, 528–530. [CrossRef]
25. Chapman, R.; Somani, B.; Robertson, A.; Healy, S.; Kata, S. Decreasing Cost of Flexible Ureterorenoscopy: Single-use Laser Fiber Cost Analysis. *Urology* **2014**, *83*, 1003–1005. [CrossRef]

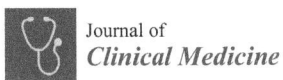

Article

Acute Kidney Injury Post-Percutaneous Nephrolithotomy (PNL): Prospective Outcomes from a University Teaching Hospital

Sunil Pillai [1], Akshay Kriplani [1], Arun Chawla [1,*], Bhaskar Somani [2], Akhilesh Pandey [3], Ravindra Prabhu [1], Anupam Choudhury [1], Shruti Pandit [1], Ravi Taori [1] and Padmaraj Hegde [1]

1. Department of Urology, Kasturba Medical College Hospital, Manipal Academy of Higher Education (MAHE), Manipal 576104, Karnataka, India; sunil.pillai@manipal.edu (S.P.); akshaykriplani@gmail.com (A.K.); ravindra.prabhu@manipal.edu (R.P.); dranupamchoudhary86@gmail.com (A.C.); shrutirpandit0492@gmail.com (S.P.); ravitaori90@gmail.com (R.T.); padmaraj.hegde@manipal.edu (P.H.)
2. Department of Urology, University Hospital Southampton NHS Trust, Southampton SO16 6YD, UK; bhaskarsomani@yahoo.com
3. Department of Community Medicine, Kasturba Medical College, Manipal Academy of Higher Education (MAHE), Manipal 576104, Karnataka, India; akhilesh.pandey@manipal.edu
* Correspondence: chawlaurology@gmail.com

Abstract: Acute Kidney Injury (AKI) after percutaneous nephrolithotomy (PNL) is a significant complication, but evidence on its incidence is bereft in the literature. The objective of this prospective observational study was to analyze the incidence of post-PNL AKI and the potential risk factors and outcomes. Demographic data collected included age, gender, body mass index (BMI), comorbidities (hypertension, diabetes mellitus), and drug history—particularly angiotensin converting enzyme inhibitors (ACE inhibitors), angiotensin II receptor blockers and beta blockers. Laboratory data included serial serum creatinine measured pre- and postoperation (12, 24, and 48 h), hemoglobin (Hb), total leucocyte count (TLC), Prothrombin time (PT), serum uric acid and urine culture. Stone factors were assessed by noncontrast computerized tomography of kidneys, ureter and bladder (NCCT KUB) and included stone burden, location and Hounsfield values. Intraoperative factors assessed were puncture site, tract size, tract number, operative time, the need for blood transfusion and stone clearance. Postoperative complications were documented using the modified Clavien–Dindo grading system and patients with postoperative AKI were followed up with serial creatinine measurements up to 1 year. Among the 509 patients analyzed, 47 (9.23%) developed postoperative AKI. Older patients, with associated hypertension and diabetes mellitus, those receiving ACE inhibitors and with lower preoperative hemoglobin and higher serum uric acid, had higher incidence of AKI. Higher stone volume and density, staghorn stones, multiple punctures and longer operative time were significantly associated with postoperative AKI. Patients with AKI had an increased length of hospital stay and 17% patients progressed to chronic kidney disease (CKD). Cut-off values for patient age (39.5 years), serum uric acid (4.05 mg/dL) and stone volume (673.06 mm^3) were assessed by receiver operating characteristic (ROC) curve analysis. Highlighting the strong predictors of post-PNL AKI allows early identification, proper counseling and postoperative planning and management in an attempt to avoid further insult to the kidney.

Keywords: acute kidney injury; percutaneous nephrolithotomy

Citation: Pillai, S.; Kriplani, A.; Chawla, A.; Somani, B.; Pandey, A.; Prabhu, R.; Choudhury, A.; Pandit, S.; Taori, R.; Hegde, P. Acute Kidney Injury Post-Percutaneous Nephrolithotomy (PNL): Prospective Outcomes from a University Teaching Hospital. *J. Clin. Med.* **2021**, *10*, 1373. https://doi.org/10.3390/jcm10071373

Academic Editor: Lee Ann MacMillan-Crow

Received: 29 January 2021
Accepted: 11 March 2021
Published: 29 March 2021

Publisher's Note: MDPI stays neutral with regard to jurisdictional claims in published maps and institutional affiliations.

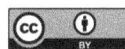

Copyright: © 2021 by the authors. Licensee MDPI, Basel, Switzerland. This article is an open access article distributed under the terms and conditions of the Creative Commons Attribution (CC BY) license (https://creativecommons.org/licenses/by/4.0/).

1. Introduction

"Primum non nocere", the preservation of renal function, is of paramount importance in the treatment of renal calculus disease, especially in view of its potential for recurrence.

Percutaneous Nephrolithotomy (PNL) is the surgical option of choice for upper urinary tract calculi with sizes of >2 cm, and selected calculi <2 cm [1]. A perceived drawback of PNL is its deleterious effect on renal function. Short- and long-term effects of PNL have been studied [2]; however, data on incidence of Acute Kidney Injury (AKI) following PNL is sparse.

Kidney Disease: Improving Global Outcomes (KDIGO) [3,4] has defined and issued practice guidelines for AKI to optimize its management [3–7]. AKI is diagnosed when one of the following criteria is met: an increase in serum creatinine greater than or equal to 0.3 mg/dL within 48 h; an increase in serum creatinine greater than or equal to 1.5 times baseline within the previous 7 days; urine volume less than or equal to 0.5 mL/kg/h for 6 h. Postoperative AKI is a significant complication in urology patients with an incidence rate of 6.7% to 38.2% [8], and is associated with poor postoperative outcomes, longer hospital stays, potential for requirement of intensive care and renal replacement therapy [5–8]. AKI-associated mortality has also been reported to be as high as 23% [9]. We have studied the incidence, risk factors and outcomes of post-PNL AKI. Postoperative complications were documented using the modified Clavien–Dindo grading system. Clinic review was at 1 month and patients with postoperative AKI were followed up with serial creatinine measurements for up to 1 year.

2. Patients and Methods

After institutional ethics committee approval and registration with the Clinical Trial registry of India (REF/2018/09/021711), we conducted a prospective observational study of consecutive patients undergoing PNL at our tertiary referral center from November 2018 to October 2019 using 4 experienced consultant endourologists. Standard PNL protocols were followed for evaluation, treatment and follow-up. Demographic data collected were age, gender, body mass index (BMI), comorbidities including hypertension, diabetes mellitus, drug history of angiotensin converting enzyme inhibitors (ACE inhibitor), angiotensin II receptor blockers and beta blockers. Laboratory data included serial serum creatinine measured pre- and postoperation (12, 24, 48 h), hemoglobin (Hb), total leucocyte count (TLC), Prothrombin time (PT), serum uric acid and urine culture. Stone factors were assessed by noncontrast computerized tomography of kidneys, ureter and bladder (NCCT KUB) and included stone burden in cubic millimeters (volume = $L \times W \times D \times \pi \times 0.167$), location and Hounsfield values and laterality. The intraoperative factors assessed were puncture site, tract size, tract number, operative time, the need for blood transfusion, stone clearance, usage of ureteral stent or nephrostomy tube and any ancillary procedures.

The operative procedure followed a standardized prone PNL protocol under general anesthesia and intravenous 3rd generation cephalosporin at induction. A sterile preoperative urine culture was ensured in all patients. All patients underwent preliminary cystoscopic insertion of a 5/6Fr ureteral catheter. Dilatation after initial puncture was carried out using serial metallic Alken dilators for conventional PNL (>24Fr) and a single-step metal dilator for the miniaturized PNL (<22Fr). The commonest tract size was 28Fr (34.8%). The irrigation fluids used during percutaneous surgery were prewarmed to body temperature in our operating room and were gravity-assisted only, with no manual pressure irrigation. Pneumatic lithotripsy, using Swiss lithoclast, was carried out for all the conventional PNLs. LASER fragmentation using a 365 μm fiber was carried out in the miniaturized PNL group. All patients had a DJ stent indwelled. Operative time was calculated from the initial puncture to final skin suture.

Postoperative blood parameters included Hb, TLC, and serum creatinine at 12, 24 and 48 h as per the clinical condition. All routine blood samples were taken at 06:00 hours. No specific diet was recommended in the immediate postoperative period. Adequate hydration was advised to all patients to maintain clear urine. Analgesia was provided using parenteral tramadol. Postoperative complications were documented using the modified Clavien–Dindo grading system [10]. This is depicted in Table 1. Patients with up to Grade 1 complications were discharged on postoperative day 2. Clinical review was at 1 month and patients with postoperative AKI were followed up with serial creatinine values up to 1 year. AKI was defined as an increase in serum creatinine ≥0.3 mg/dL within 48 h. Chronic Kidney Disease (CKD) was defined by an estimated glomerular filtration rate (eGFR) of <60 mL/min/1.73 m². eGFR was calculated by using the four variable Modification of Diet in Renal Disease (MDRD) formula.

Table 1. Clavien–Dindo complications after percutaneous nephrolithotomy (PNL): $n = 517$.

Complication	Clavien–Dindo	15Fr	22Fr	24Fr	26Fr	28Fr	30Fr	32Fr	34Fr	36Fr	p-Value
Fever	2	8	0	3	8	18	4	12	1	2	0.743
Haematuria	1	0	0	2	5	3	1	8	0	0	0.342
Angioembolization	3B	0	0	1	3	2	0	0	0	0	0.663
Auxiliary proc.											0.143
URS		0	0	0	2	3	1	1	0	0	
2nd PNL		0	0	0	2	0	0	2	0	0	
Bladder wash		0	0	1	2	0	0	2	0	0	
Stent reposition	3A	0	0	0	0	0	1	0	0	0	
Visual internal Urethrotomy		0	0	0	0	0	0	0	0	1	

URS: Ureterorenoscopy.

Statistical analysis was carried out on SPSS, Version 16.0. Categorical variables are expressed in frequencies with percentages and were compared using Chi-square or Fisher's exact test. Continuous variables with normal distributions are expressed as mean and standard deviation and were compared using Student's t-test; those with skewed distributions are expressed as medians and interquartile range with comparison using Mann–Whitney test; a p-value ≤ 0.05 was considered significant. Univariate analysis was carried out to assess the relation between the dependent variable (occurrence of AKI) and each of the independent variables. Multivariate analysis was then performed using logistic regression to establish the predictive factors for the development of AKI. A receiver operating characteristic (ROC) curve was constructed, and a value of area under the curve above 0.65 was considered a cut-off value for the variable.

3. Results

Of 517 patients, 8 (1.5%) who had preoperative AKI were excluded (Figure 1). There were no patients with a solitary kidney in this study. All patients had normal contralateral kidneys. Three patients had a history of previous PNL in the ipsilateral unit, and one patient had history of PNL in the contralateral unit. No other renal procedures were noted in other patients. Of the remaining 509, the mean age was 48.1 ± 13.92, with 388 (76.2%) males and 121 (23.8%) females. Ninety-four (18.5%) and 142 (27.9%) patients had diabetes Mellitus and hypertension, respectively, and 47 (9.23%) developed postoperative AKI.

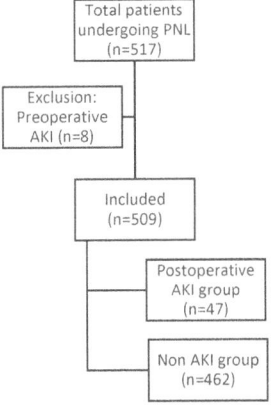

Figure 1. Flow chart of patients during the study period. AKI-Acute Kidney Injury; PNL-Percutaneous Nephrolithotomy.

Details of patient demographics and stone characteristics with the univariate analysis for independent predictive factors for development of postoperative AKI are mentioned in Tables 2–4. Those with AKI were older (mean age 54.8 ± 13.9 vs. 47.4 ± 13.7 years, OR = 1.041, 95% CI = 1.017–1.066, p = 0.001), significantly more likely to have hypertension (51.1% vs. 25.5%, OR = 3.042, 95% CI = 1.655–5.593, p = 0.0002), diabetes mellitus (29.8% vs. 17.3%, OR = 2.026, 95% CI = 1.037–3.959, p = 0.036), have received ACE inhibitors (10.6% vs. 3.7%, OR = 3.116, 95% CI = 1.095–8.871, p = 0.036), have lower preoperative hemoglobin (12.6 ± 2.25 vs. 13.3 ± 1.86, p = 0.013) and have higher serum uric acid (5.2 ± 1.46 vs. 3.9 ± 1.44, OR = 1.758, 95% CI = 1.336–2.315, p = 0.00001) as compared to those without AKI. Stone volume (mm^3) (2117.9 (761–12,452) vs. 825 (503–1573) p = 0.0000001), stone density (817.4 ± 439.76 vs. 985.2 ± 253.98, p = 0.0001) and number of staghorn stones (12.8% vs. 3.2%, OR = 4.361, 95% CI = 1.605–11.846, p = 0.008) were significant higher in those with AKI.

Table 2. Patient characteristics, preoperative laboratory values and stone characteristics.

Variables		All Patients (n = 509)	AKI Cohort (n = 47)	Non-AKI (n = 462)	p-Value
Patient Characteristics					
Age (years) (mean ± SD)		48.13 ± 13.92	54.83 ± 13.907	47.45 ± 13.75	0.001
Gender (M)		388 (76.2%)	39 (83%)	349 (75.5%)	0.254
Gender (F)		121 (23.8%)	8 (17%)	113 (24.5%)	
BMI (kg/m^2)		25.23 ± 2.94	25.21 ± 3.12	25.23 ± 2.92	0.974
Hypertension		142 (27.9%)	24 (51.1%)	118 (25.5%)	0.0002
Diabetes mellitus		94 (18.5%)	14 (29.8%)	80 (17.3%)	0.036
ACE inhibitors		22 (4.3%)	5 (10.6%)	17 (3.7%)	0.043
Beta-blockers		10 (2%)	1 (2.1%)	9 (1.9%)	1.00
Preoperative Laboratory Values					
Hemoglobin (mg/dL)		13.29 ± 1.91	12.63 ± 2.25	13.36 ± 1.86	0.013
Platelet(/μL)		273,669.36 ± 79,821.98	276,833.33 ± 103,392.68	273,354 ± 77,278.68	0.778
Prothrombin time (s)		10.58 ± 0.39	10.75 ± 0.66	10.55 ± 0.32	0.006
Creatinine (mg/dL)		1.42 ± 4.30	1.34 ± 0.76	1.43 ± 4.5	0.895
Uric Acid (mg/dL)		4.13 ± 1.52	5.23 ± 1.46	3.91 ± 1.44	0.00001
Total leucocyte count (/mm^3)		8.73 ± 3.84	9.73 ± 9.54	8.63 ± 2.65	0.06
Stone Characteristics					
Stone Volume (mm^3) (median (Q1–Q3))		880.95 (524.38–1801.25)	2117.94 (761–12,452)	825 (503–1573)	0.00
Hounsfield Unit (HU)		970.59 ± 278.55	817.45 ± 439.76	985.18 ± 253.98	0.0001
Stone location	Upper Calyx	26 (5.1%)	2 (4.3%)	24 (5.2%)	1.000
	Middle Calyx	53 (10.4%)	9 (19.1%)	44 (9.5%)	0.074
	Lower Calyx	138 (27.1%)	15 (31.9%)	123 (26.6%)	0.437
	Pelvic	190 (37.3%)	14 (29.8%)	176 (38.1%)	0.262
	PUJ	153 (30.1%)	12 (25.5%)	141 (30.5%)	0.477
	Staghorn	21 (4.12%)	6 (12.8%)	15 (3.24%)	0.008

ACE, Angiotensin converting enzyme; PUJ, Pelvi-ureteric junction.

Table 3. Intraoperative data.

Variables		All Patients (n = 509)	AKI Cohort (n = 47)	Non-AKI (n = 462)	p
Puncture site	Supracostal	75 (14.7%)	5 (10.6%)	70 (15.2%)	0.406
	Infracostal	434 (85.3%)	42 (89.4%)	392 (84.8%)	
Tract size (Fr) (median (Q1–Q3))		28 (26–32)	28 (26–28)	28 (26–32)	0.032
Puncture Number	Single Puncture	497 (97.6%)	43 (91.5%)	454 (98.3%)	0.019
	>1 Puncture	12 (2.35%)	4 (8.51%)	8 (1.73%)	
Blood Transfusion		15 (2.9%)	3 (6.4%)	12 (2.6%)	0.153
Operative time (minutes)		55.99 ± 16.71	63.51 ± 21.79	55.23 ± 15.93	0.001

Table 4. Univariate and multivariate logistic regression analyses for predictors of post-PNL Acute Kidney Injury (AKI).

Variable		Univariate Analysis		Multivariate Analysis	
		Unadjusted OR	p-Value	Adjusted OR	p-Value
Age		1.041 (1.017–1.066)	0.001	1.050 (0.998–1.105)	0.060
Gender	Male	1.578 (0.717–3.477)	0.257	0.129 (0.021–0.787)	0.026
	Female	1.0		1.0	
BMI		0.998 (0.901–1.106)	0.974	0.712 (0.550–0.923)	0.010
Hypertension	Yes	3.042 (1.655–5.593)	0.0003	2.514 (0.699–9.035)	0.158
	No	1.0		1.0	
Diabetes Mellitus	Yes	2.026 (1.037–3.959)	0.039	2.423 (0.521–11.260)	0.259
	No	1.0		1.0	
ACE inhibitors	Yes	3.116 (1.095–8.871)	0.033	60.404 (1.619–2253.49)	0.026
	No	1.0		1.0	
Beta-blocker	Yes	1.094 (0.136–8.830)	0.933	0.770 (0.031–19.033)	0.873
	No	1.0		1.0	
Creatinine		0.994 (0.911–1.085)	0.896	1.332 (0.861–2.059)	0.198
Uric Acid		1.758 (1.336–2.315)	0.00005	2.163 (1.459–3.209)	0.0001
Total leucocyte count		1.045 (0.989–1.103)	0.116	0.999 (0.841–1.187)	0.988
Operative Time		1.028 (0.983–1.049)	0.001	1.015 (0.982–1.049)	0.364
Blood Transfusion (n)	Yes	2.557 (0.695–9.405)	0.158	8.408 (0.396–178.42)	0.172
	No	1.0		1.0	
Stone size		1.000		1.000	
Stone Location (n)	Upper calyx	0.811 (0.186–3.545)	0.781	0.223 (0.011–4.509)	0.328
	Middle calyx	2.250 (1.021–4.959)	0.044	1.822 (0.269–12.370)	0.539
	Lower calyx	1.292 (0.676–2.467)	0.438	1.843 (0.336–10.121)	0.482
	Pelvis	0.689 (0.359–1.324)	0.264	1.897 (0.333–10.796)	0.471
	PUJ	0.478 (0.394–1.548)	0.781	1.582 (0.205–12.207)	0.660
	Staghorn	4.361 (1.605–11.846)	0.004	0.594 (0.032–10.944)	0.726
Tract number (n)	Single Tract	1.000		1.000	
	>1 Tracts	5.279 (1.527–18.248)	0.009	89.698 (0.795–10,119.9)	0.062
Tract site (n)	Supracostal	0.667 (0.255–1.744)	0.408	0.054 (0.003–1.121)	0.05
	Infracostal				

(OR—Odds Ratio).

Among operative characteristics (Table 3), those with AKI had a significantly greater number of punctures (8.5% vs. 1.7%, OR = 5.279, 95% CI = 1.527–18.248, $p = 0.019$) and longer operative time (63.5 ± 21.8 vs. 55.2 ± 15.9 min, OR = 1.028, 95% CI = 0.983–1.049, $p = 0.001$). Forty-five patients in the AKI group had complete stone clearance with a stone free rate (SFR) of 95.7%. None of our patients had persistent intraoperative or postoperative hypotension requiring inotropic support. In total, two patients underwent selective angioembolization in our study.

Multivariable logistic regression analysis further demonstrated that factors significantly associated with postoperative AKI were gender (male, OR = 0.129, 95% CI = 0.021–0.787, $p = 0.026$), BMI (OR = 0.712, 95% CI = 0.550–0.923, $p = 0.010$), use of ACE inhibitors (OR = 60.404, 95% CI = 1.619–2253.49, $p = 0.026$) serum uric acid (OR = 2.163, 95% CI = 1.459–3.209, $p = 0.0001$) and puncture site (OR = 0.054, 95% CI = 0.003–1.121, $p = 0.059$). Prothrombin time and tract size were found to not be statistically significant in the preliminary analysis and were excluded from the subsequent univariate and multivariate analyses. All other variables were included.

The ROC curve was built for the variables, including age, serum uric acid and stone volume, to better define the independent predictive ability of the variables that were clinically and statistically important in both the univariate and multivariate analyses. ROC analysis was carried out to generate a cut-off value that would be informative for urologists to decide on intensive care unit (ICU) requirement and prognosis. In the ROC analysis, patients with ages greater than 39.5 years had 81% sensitivity and 26.9% specificity; those with serum uric acid levels greater than 4.05 mg/dL had 90.1% sensitivity and 55.2% specificity, with an area under curve of 79.1%; those with stone volume greater than 673.06 mm^3 had 90.5% sensitivity and 46.3% specificity and area under curve of 70.7%; these were all associated with development of AKI. Three (6.38%) patients required postoperative hemodialysis in view of oliguria and hyperkalemia. Two of these patients required two sessions for clinical recovery, whereas the third patient recovered after a single session. Among the AKI cohort, the mean creatinine values preoperation, immediately postoperation, at the time of discharge and at the one-year follow-up were 1.3 ± 0.766, 1.3 ± 0.99, 5.05 ± 22.01 and 1.7 ± 1.12, respectively. Serum creatinine was significantly higher by 0.249 mg/dL ($p = 0.010$, 95% CI = 0.063–0.435) at one year as compared to postoperative values and eight patients (17.02%) in the AKI group progressed to CKD at the 1 year follow-up.

4. Discussion

Renal function can be affected by stone disease or obstruction related to it, urinary infections and by surgical intervention. Though the intent of treatment is to improve renal function, it is plausible that it could have an adverse effect. The risk of impairment exists for all levels of invasiveness—from SWL (elvi-ureteric junction.) to URS (Ureterorenoscopy) and PNL (Percutaneous Nephrolithotomy). The choice of treatment depends on stone factors, patient factors including comorbidities, surgical expertise, and also underlying renal function. A systematic review by Reeves et al. suggests that the overall renal function is not always detrimentally affected by endourological interventions [2]. Morbidities after PNL such as fever, bleeding, pleural or visceral injury and significant nephron loss have been well described [11]. Incidence of postoperative AKI for major open urological procedures varies from 6.7% to 38.2% [5–9]. Surprisingly, very few studies report complications of PNL and AKI [12–14]. This may be because impairment of renal function in the absence of significant perioperative complications appears to be minimal, transient and focal. Effect on renal function is influenced by preoperative renal status and presence of comorbidities such as diabetes mellitus and hypertension [15]. Violation of the renal parenchyma, high irrigation pressure, tract multiplicity, preoperative urine infection and postoperative bleeding are reported as attributes causing post-PNL AKI [2,16]. However, subsequent improvement in renal function is seen in almost all renal units that are obstructed and infected [15,17]. Standardized definition of AKI was introduced to aid early detection and management and improve the overall patient outcomes [3]. As AKI may be associated with mortality in up to 23% patients [9], with increased duration of hospital stay and requirement of intensive care, every attempt should be made to identify predisposing factors and predictors of postoperative AKI.

In our prospective study, we found an incidence of post-PNL AKI of 9.2%, which was comparable to incidence reported in the literature [5–9]. We divided the AKI predictors into patient factors, stone factors and operative factors. Patient factors associated with a higher risk for AKI were older age, presence of comorbidities such as hypertension and diabetes mellitus, and preoperative use of ACE inhibitors or angiotensin II inhibitors, which may be due to loss of renal reserve or decreased glomerular filtration rate (GFR) due to these factors.

Reduced plasma volume, cardiac and neuronal changes, leading to intraoperative hypotension in elderly patients, are described as causing postoperative AKI [13,18]. Autonomic neuropathy due to diabetes is known to cause perioperative hemodynamic changes [19]. Persistent hypotension in the postoperative period leads to deterioration of renal function. None of our patients had persistent intraoperative or postoperative hypotension requiring inotropic support. Alteration in the renin angiotensin system due to use of ACE inhibitors or angiotensin II inhibitors is a known predisposing factor for renal hypoperfusion, as was seen in 10.6% of patients with AKI in our cohort, making these drugs an independent predictor of AKI [20]. Low hemoglobin and leukocytosis were predictive of post-PNL AKI in our study.

The lack of evidence in the literature makes it difficult to explain the correlation of low hemoglobin with postoperative AKI, but infection related leukocytosis may affect AKI by affecting inflammatory mediators in microcirculation. High serum uric acid levels are another risk factor for AKI, in agreement with other reported studies [21]. Crystal-independent mechanisms and crystal-dependent pathways are postulated for this. High serum uric acid can induce renal vasoconstriction and impair autoregulation, which results in reduced renal blood flow and GFR. The proposed mechanism responsible is the activation of proinflammatory cascade leading to endothelial dysfunction, which causes impaired autoregulation and renal vasoconstriction [21–23]. High serum uric acid levels could therefore be potentially used to help identify patients at high risk of developing AKI [21].

Stone factors such a high stone volume, density and staghorn calculi increases the complexity of the procedure and operative time, with increased risk of perioperative bleeding and infective complications, leading to AKI [14,23]. These may serve as surrogate markers for development of AKI as also observed in our study.

Literature evidence suggests multiple tracts and larger tract size causes significant nephron damage and leads to AKI [14,24–26]. However, we did not find tract size to be an independent significant factor in this study. Though no morphological or functional decline by imaging and nuclear studies at the access site has been studied in the literature, it can be interpreted that the presence of multiple tracts and larger tracts cause cellular injury. Emerging urinary biomarkers such as neutrophil gelatinase-associated lipocalin (NGAL), predictive of ischemic AKI or AKI in transplant kidney after renal biopsy, have been reported in the literature [27]. In our study, cut-off values of age (39.5 years), serum uric acid (4.05 mg/dL) and stone volume (673.06 mm^3) showed high sensitivity to predict postoperative AKI.

AKI commonly leads to increased length of hospital stay [12,28]. In our study, the mean length of hospitalization was not increased in the AKI group due to a lack of clinical deterioration in this cohort of patients. The majority were therefore managed conservatively, while 6.38% patients required renal replacement therapy. However, progression to CKD can be a sequelae of AKI [29], although complete improvement in renal function after 6–12 months has also been reported [14,30,31]. In our study, 17.02% patients in the AKI cohort progressed to CKD.

A large sample size and medium-term follow-up provided strength to this study, highlighting the strong predictors of post-PNL AKI. Counseling and postoperative planning in consultation with nephrology, avoidance of nephrotoxic drugs and appropriate fluid management are key to avoiding further insult to the kidney. Lack of a control group testing against other interventions and a urolithiasis scoring system for percutaneous nephrolithotomy outcomes, such as the Guy's scoring system, are limitations of our study.

5. Conclusions

Up to 10% patients can develop post-PNL AKI, of which one-fifth can progress to CKD. Older age, presence of hypertension, diabetes mellitus, low hemoglobin, leukocytosis, high uric acid levels, staghorn calculi, use of multiple tracts and longer operative times all predict the development of AKI. Highlighting the strong predictors of post-PNL AKI allows early identification, proper counseling and postoperative planning in an attempt to avoid further insult to the kidney and care must be taken to optimize these conditions to minimize AKI.

Author Contributions: Concept and Study design: A.C. (Arun Chawla), A.K. and S.P. (Sunil Pillai); Methods and experimental work: A.C. (Arun Chawla), A.K., S.P. (Shruti Pandit), P.H. and S.P. (Sunil Pillai); Results analysis and conclusions: A.C. (Arun Chawla), A.C. (Anupam Choudhury), A.P., R.P., R.T. and S.P. (Sunil Pillai); Manuscript preparation: A.K., S.P. (Sunil Pillai), R.P. and B.S. All authors have read and agreed to the published version of the manuscript.

Funding: This research received no external funding.

Institutional Review Board Statement: Institutional ethics committee approval: 477/2018. Clinical Trial registry of India (REF/2018/09/021711).

Informed Consent Statement: Informed consent was obtained from all subjects involved in the study.

Data Availability Statement: NA.

Conflicts of Interest: The authors declare no conflict of interest.

References

1. Türk, C.; Petřík, A.; Sarica, K.; Seitz, C.; Skolarikos, A.; Straub, M.; Knoll, T. EAU guidelines on interventional treatment for urolithiasis. *Eur. Urol.* **2016**, *69*, 475–482. [CrossRef]
2. Reeves, T.; Pietropaolo, A.; Gadzhiev, N.; Seitz, C.; Somani, B.K. Role of Endourological Procedures (PCNL and URS) on Renal Function: A Systematic Review. *Curr. Urol. Rep.* **2020**, *21*, 21. [CrossRef]
3. Mehta, R.L.; Kellum, J.A.; Shah, S.V.; Molitoris, B.A.; Ronco, C.; Warnock, D.G.; Levin, A. Acute Kidney Injury Network: Report of an initiative to improve outcomes in acute kidney injury. *Crit. Care* **2007**, *11*, R31. [CrossRef]
4. Kidney Disease: Improving Global Outcomes (KDIGO) Acute Kidney Injury Work Group. KDIGO Clinical Practice Guideline for Acute Kidney Injury. *Kidney Int. Suppl.* **2012**, *2*, 1–138.
5. Chertow, G.M.; Burdick, E.; Honour, M.; Bonventre, J.V.; Bates, D.W. Acute kidney injury, mortality, length of stay, and costs in hospitalized patients. *J. Am. Soc. Nephrol.* **2005**, *16*, 3365–3370. [CrossRef] [PubMed]
6. Hobson, C.; Ozrazgat-Baslanti, T.; Kuxhausen, A.; Thottakkara, P.; Efron, P.A.; Moore, F.A.; Moldawer, L.L.; Segal, M.S.; Bihorac, A. Cost and mortality associated with postoperative acute kidney injury. *Ann. Surg.* **2015**, *261*, 1207–1214. [CrossRef] [PubMed]
7. Okusa, M.D.; Davenport, A. Reading between the (guide) lines: The KD IGO practice guideline on acute kidney injury in the individual patient. *Kidney Int.* **2014**, *85*, 39–48. [CrossRef]
8. Caddeo, G.; Williams, S.T.; McIntyre, C.W.; Selby, N.M. Acute kidney injury in urology patients: Incidence, causes and outcomes. *Nephrourol. Mon.* **2013**, *5*, 955–961. [CrossRef] [PubMed]
9. Thongprayoon, C.; Cheungpasitporn, W.; Akhoundi, A.; Ahmed, A.H.; Kashani, K.B. Actual versus ideal body weight for acute kidney injury diagnosis and classification in critically Ill patients. *BMC Nephrol.* **2014**, *15*, 176. [CrossRef]
10. De La Rosette, J.J.; Opondo, D.; Daels, F.P.; Giusti, G.; Serrano, A.; Kandasami, S.V.; Wolf, J.S., Jr.; Grabe, M.; Gravas, S.; Croes Pcnl Study Group. Categorisation of complications and validation of the Clavien score for percutaneous nephrolithotomy. *Eur. Urol.* **2012**, *62*, 246–255. [CrossRef] [PubMed]
11. Michel, M.S.; Trojan, L.; Rassweiler, J.J. Complications in percutaneous nephrolithotomy. *Eur. Urol.* **2007**, *51*, 899–906, discussion 906. [CrossRef]
12. Yu, J.; Park, H.K.; Kwon, H.J.; Lee, J.; Hwang, J.H.; Kim, H.Y. Risk factors for acute kidney injury after percutaneous nephrolithotomy: Implications of intraoperative hypotension. *Medicine* **2018**, *97*, e11580. [CrossRef]
13. Fulla, J.; Calle, J.; Elia, M.; Wright, H.; Li, I. MP22-03 Acute kidney injury and percutaneous nephrolithotomy: Frequency and predictive factors. *J. Urol.* **2020**, *203* (Suppl. 4), e328. [CrossRef]

14. El-Nahas, A.R.; Taha, D.E.; Ali, H.M.; Elshal, A.M.; Zahran, M.H.; El-Tabey, N.A.; El-Assmy, A.M.; Harraz, A.M.; Moawad, H.E.; Othman, M.M. Othman Acute kidney injury after percutaneous nephrolithotomy for stones in solitary kidneys. *Scand. J. Urol.* **2017**, *51*, 165–169. [CrossRef]
15. Patel, R.; Agarwal, S.; Sankhwar, S.N.; Goel, A.; Singh, B.P.; Kumar, M. A prospective study assessing feasibility of performing percutaneous nephrolithotomy in chronic kidney disease patients—What factors affect the outcome? *Int. Braz J. Urol.* **2019**, *45*, 765–774. [CrossRef]
16. Emiliani, E.; Talso, M.; Baghdadi, M.; Traxer, O. Renal parenchyma injury after percutaneous nephrolithotomy tract dilatations in pig and cadaveric kidney models. *Cent. Eur. J. Urol.* **2017**, *70*, 69–75.
17. Sairam, K.; Scoffone, C.M.; Alken, P.; Turna, B. Percutaneous nephrolithotomy and chronic kidney disease: Results from the CROES PC NL Global Study. *J. Urol.* **2012**, *188*, 1195–1200. [CrossRef] [PubMed]
18. Charlson, M.E.; MacKenzie, C.R.; Gold, J.P.; Ales, K.L.; Topkins, M.; Shires, G.T. Preoperative characteristics predicting intraoperative hypotension and hypertension among hypertensives and diabetics undergoing noncardiac surgery. *Ann. Surg.* **1990**, *212*, 66–81. [CrossRef]
19. Oakley, I.; Emond, L. Diabetic cardiac autonomic neuropathy and anesthetic management: Review of the literature. *AANA J.* **2011**, *79*, 473–479.
20. Comfere, T.; Sprung, J.; Kumar, M.M.; Draper, M.; Wilson, D.P.; Williams, B.A.; Danielson, D.R.; Liedl, L.; Warner, D.O. Angiotensin system inhibitors in a general surgical population. *Anesth Analg.* **2005**, *100*, 636–644. [CrossRef]
21. Cheungpasitporn, W.; Thongprayoon, C.; Harrison, A.M.; Erickson, S.B. Admission hyperuricemia increases the risk of acute kidney injury in hospitalized patients. *Clin. Kidney J.* **2016**, *9*, 51–56. [CrossRef]
22. Ejaz, A.A.; Johnson, R.J.; Shimada, M.; Mohandas, R.; Alquadan, K.F.; Beaver, T.M.; Lapsia, V.; Dass, B. The Role of Uric Acid in Acute Kidney Injury. *Nephron* **2019**, *142*, 275–283. [CrossRef]
23. De la Rosette, J.J.; Zuazu, J.R.; Tsakiris, P.; Elsakka, A.M.; Zudaire, J.J.; Laguna, M.P.; de Reijke, T.M. Prognostic factors and percutaneous nephrolithotomy morbidity: A multivariate analysis of a contemporary series using the Clavien classification. *J. Urol.* **2008**, *180*, 2489–2493. [CrossRef]
24. Muslumanoglu, A.Y.; Tefekli, A.; Karadag, M.A.; Tok, A.; Sari, E.; Berberoglu, Y. Impact of percutaneous access point number and location on complication and success rates in percutaneous nephrolithotomy. *Urol. Int.* **2006**, *77*, 340–346. [CrossRef]
25. Aron, M.; Yadav, R.; Goel, R.; Kolla, S.B.; Gautam, G.; Hemal, A.K.; Gupta, N.P. Multi-tract percutaneous nephrolithotomy for large complete staghorn calculi. *Urol. Int.* **2005**, *75*, 327–332. [CrossRef]
26. Rashid, A.O.; Fakhulddin, S.S. Risk factors for fever and sepsis after percutaneous nephrolithotomy. *Asian J. Urol.* **2016**, *3*, 82–87. [CrossRef]
27. Devarajan, P. Emerging urinary biomarkers in the diagnosis of acute kidney injury. *Expert Opin. Med. Diagn.* **2008**, *2*, 387–398. [CrossRef] [PubMed]
28. Borthwick, E.; Ferguson, A. Perioperative acute kidney injury: Risk factors, recognition, management, and outcomes. *BMJ* **2010**, *341*, c3365. [CrossRef] [PubMed]
29. Venkatachalam, M.A.; Griffin, K.A.; Lan, R.; Geng, H.; Saikumar, P.; Bidani, A.K. Acute kidney injury: A springboard for progression in chronic kidney disease. *Am. J. Physiol. Renal. Physiol.* **2010**, *298*, F1078–F1094. [CrossRef]
30. Bucuras, V.; Gopalakrishnam, G.; Wolf, J.S., Jr.; Sun, Y.; Bianchi, G.; Erdogru, T.; de la Rosette, on behalf of the CROES PCNL Study Group. The Clinical Research Office of the Endourological Society Percutaneous Nephrolithotomy Global Study: Nephrolithotomy in 189 patients with solitary kidneys. *J. Endourol.* **2012**, *26*, 336–341. [CrossRef] [PubMed]
31. Shi, X.; Peng, Y.; Li, L.; Li, X.; Wang, Q.; Zhang, W.; Dong, H.; Shen, R.; Lu, C.; Liu, M.; et al. Renal function changes after percutaneous nephrolithotomy in patients with renal calculi with a solitary kidney compared to bilateral kidneys. *BJU Int.* **2018**, *122*, 633–638. [CrossRef] [PubMed]

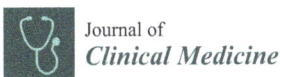

Article

Risk of Metabolic Syndrome in Kidney Stone Formers: A Comparative Cohort Study with a Median Follow-Up of 19 Years

Robert M. Geraghty [1], Paul Cook [2], Paul Roderick [3] and Bhaskar Somani [4],*

[1] Department of Urology, Freeman Hospital, Newcastle-upon-Tyne NE7 7DN, UK; rob.geraghty@newcastle.ac.uk
[2] Department of Biochemistry, University Hospital Southampton, Southampton SO16 6YD, UK; Paul.Cook@uhs.nhs.uk
[3] Department of Public Health, University of Southampton, Southampton SO16 6YD, UK; pjr@soton.ac.uk
[4] Department of Urology, University Hospital Southampton, Southampton SO16 6YD, UK
* Correspondence: bhaskarsomani@yahoo.com; Tel.: +44-023-807-772-22

Citation: Geraghty, R.M.; Cook, P.; Roderick, P.; Somani, B. Risk of Metabolic Syndrome in Kidney Stone Formers: A Comparative Cohort Study with a Median Follow-Up of 19 Years. *J. Clin. Med.* **2021**, *10*, 978. https://doi.org/10.3390/jcm10050978

Academic Editor: Wisit Cheungpasitporn

Received: 30 January 2021
Accepted: 18 February 2021
Published: 2 March 2021

Publisher's Note: MDPI stays neutral with regard to jurisdictional claims in published maps and institutional affiliations.

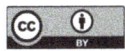

Copyright: © 2021 by the authors. Licensee MDPI, Basel, Switzerland. This article is an open access article distributed under the terms and conditions of the Creative Commons Attribution (CC BY) license (https://creativecommons.org/licenses/by/4.0/).

Abstract: Background: Kidney stone formers (SF) are more likely to develop diabetes mellitus (DM), but there is no study examining risk of metabolic syndrome (MetS) in this population. We aimed to describe the risk of MetS in SF compared to non-SF. Methods and Materials: SF referred to a tertiary referral metabolic centre in Southern England from 1990 to 2007, comparator patients were age, sex, and period (first stone) matched with 3:1 ratio from the same primary care database. SF with no documentation or previous MetS were excluded. Ethical approval was obtained and MetS was defined using the modified Association of American Clinical Endocrinologists (AACE) criteria. Analysis with cox proportional hazard regression. Results: In total, 828 SF were included after 1000 records were screened for inclusion, with 2484 age and sex matched non-SF comparators. Median follow-up was 19 years (interquartile range—IQR: 15–22) for both stone formers and stone-free comparators. SF were at significantly increased risk of developing MetS (hazard ratio—HR: 1.77; 95% confidence interval—CI: 1.55–2.03, $p < 0.001$). This effect was robust to adjustment for pre-existing components (HR: 1.91; 95% CI: 1.66–2.19, $p < 0.001$). Conclusions: Kidney stone formers are at increased risk of developing metabolic syndrome. Given the pathophysiological mechanism, the stone is likely a 'symptom' of an underlying metabolic abnormality, whether covert or overt. This has implications the risk of further stone events and cardiovascular disease.

Keywords: kidney stones; metabolic syndrome; urolithiasis; nephrolithiasis; kidney calculi; diabetes mellitus

1. Introduction

Kidney stone disease (KSD) is a costly [1] and increasingly prevalent problem, with the latest USA prevalence (2015–2016) being 10% [2]. Amongst the risk factors for development of KSD, type 2 diabetes mellitus and the metabolic syndrome (MetS) [3] are particularly well described. Both are characterised by high blood glucose and insulin resistance [4] and share common pathophysiologic mechanisms that attributes to the increased risk of KSD, e.g., urinary acidification [5]. This translates to a proportional increase in uric acid stones [6]. Given the MetS pandemic [7], this will lead to worldwide increases in KSD.

The other components of MetS (obesity, hypertension and dyslipidaemia) have all been described, to varying degrees, as carrying increased risk of KSD. There is good epidemiological evidence for the link between obesity and an associated risk of KSD [8]. However, the cause of this increased risk is likely due to the metabolic sequelae of obesity, such as dyslipidaemia and insulin resistance [5].

There is conflicting evidence for the risk of KSD in hypertensives. Unadjusted crude risk demonstrates significantly increased risk of hypertensives becoming stone formers [9,10]. However, on adjustment the increased risk is rendered non-significant [9,10]. This is likely due to the confounding presence of other KSD risk factors, e.g., high blood glucose or dyslipidaemia.

Dyslipidaemia (high serum triglycerides and low high-density lipoprotein) causes demonstrable derangements in 24 h urinary biochemistries [11]. A further sequela of dyslipidaemia is lipotoxicity (abnormal lipid accumulation in tissues) [12]. In the kidney, lipotoxicity reduces ammonium secretion and lowers pH (both risk factors for KSD) [11].

Not only are the components of MetS risk factors for KSD, the reverse is also true. Stone formers are at increased risk of developing both diabetes mellitus [13] and hypertension [14]. As yet however, there is no evidence for increased risk of MetS in stone formers.

The importance of a MetS diagnosis is the increased risk of cardiovascular disease [15]. Although the definition has changed over the years, the consensus across multiple large cohort studies is a 2- to 4-fold increase in risk of cardiovascular disease in those with MetS. This has clinical implications for individuals and populations.

As there has been no study examining the risk of developing MetS in the stone forming population, our primary aim was to describe this risk in stone formers. Our secondary aims were to examine the risk of individual MetS components and risk of MetS per stone type.

2. Methods

2.1. Definitions

Metabolic syndrome was defined using the Association of American Clinical Endocrinologists (AACE) criteria [4], which is similar to the more widely used National Cholesterol Education Program Adult Treatment Panel (NCEP ATP) III criteria. It replaces waist circumference with (body mass index) BMI > 25, as waist circumference was not available on electronic records. In addition to AACE criteria, specific treatment for hyperglycaemia or hypertension were included, as well as physician diagnosis (see Table 1). Development of three or more components was defined as incident Metabolic syndrome (MetS). Age of development of MetS defined as age at which 3 or more components present, components assumed to be cumulative, i.e., patients will not lose diabetic or hypertensive, etc., status with increasing age.

Electronic records included all clinical letters, operation notes, test results, diagnoses, treatments, and basic readings including blood pressure, height, and weight.

Table 1. Metabolic syndrome definition.

Metabolic Syndrome (Modified AACE Criteria)	
Fasting Plasma Glucose	>6.1 mmol/L or Hypoglycaemic treatment or Physician diagnosis of Impaired Glucose Tolerance or Diabetes Mellitus
Body Mass Index	≥ 25 kg/m^2 or Physician diagnosis of Obesity
Blood Pressure	$\geq 130/\geq 85$ mmHg or Antihypertensive treatment or Physician diagnosis of hypertension
Triglycerides	>1.7 mmol/L
High-Density Lipoprotein	M: <1.04 mmol/L; F: <1.29 mmol/L

2.2. Study Population

The cohort consisted of patients with kidney stone disease (KSD) presenting to a tertiary referral hospital referred for metabolic assessment between 1990 and 2007. The study population has been described in a previous cross-sectional study [16] and subsequent cohort study [1]. During this period, stone formers were routinely referred to this clinic by the urology team (both in Southampton and around the region—Dorset, Wiltshire, and Hampshire) and general practitioners. In total, 1000 (from 2801) patients were selected by block randomization after alphabetization of surnames.

Further information on past medical history and subsequent stone recurrence was ascertained retrospectively using hospital and general practice electronic records. The general practice electronic records is downloaded to the Care and Health Information Exchange (CHIE), a large database including data from 172 general practices within Hampshire and the Isle of Wight (95% coverage).

Data collected in retrospect using CHIE: age, sex, past medical history at first presentation, including metabolic syndrome components (see Table 1) and incident metabolic syndrome components. Subsequent stone episodes and stone type were ascertained using a combination of CHIE and hospital records. See Appendix A for stone disease read codes.

Patients who had no documentation (i.e., no evidence of subsequent follow-up or consultation, lived outside or have left Hampshire, or no documentation on CHIE) or had pre-existing metabolic syndrome (MetS) were excluded (see Figure 1).

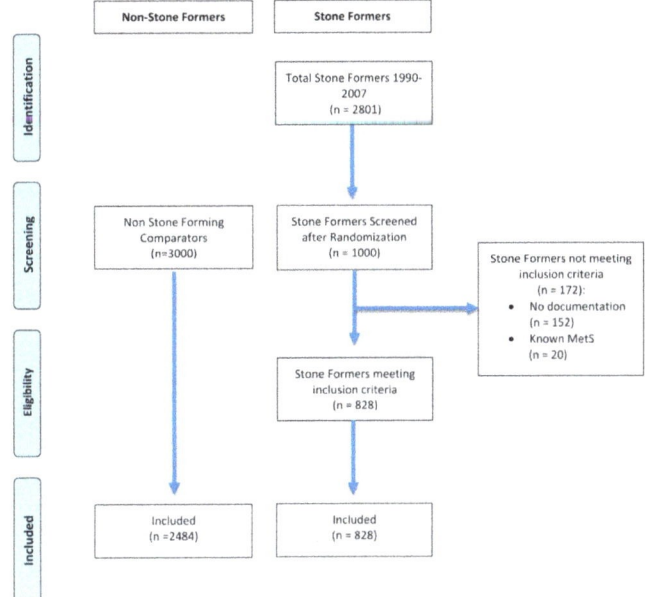

Figure 1. CONSORT flow diagram of patient selection.

2.3. Comparator Population

Comparator data was supplied by Care and Health Information Analytics (CHIA), the body utilising CHIE data for research, using age (within 5 years), sex, and region matched patients in a ratio of 3:1 once stone formers (SF) had been screened for eligibility. The follow-up period was matched as closely as possible.

Patients with codes associated with KSD (see Appendix A) and previous components of metabolic syndrome were excluded. Data on incident metabolic syndrome components were collected (see Table 1), time defined as initial age to age at which first reached diagnostic criteria for metabolic syndrome component.

Only practices which were present within CHIA on 1st May 2019 were selected to be included. Random patients were selected from this practice cohort. Data on age of development of MetS components and death (if applicable) were extracted.

2.4. Statistical Methods

SPSS (version 26, IBM, Armonk, NY, USA) and R statistical package version 3.6.3 (R Foundation for Statistical Computing, Vienna, Austria. URL https://www.R-project.org/) (packages: survival and survminer) were used for statistical analysis. Cox proportional hazards model was used to analyse the data, which is presented as hazard ratio (HR) with 95% confidence interval (CI). Time to event was defined as time from presentation to metabolic stone clinic to development of 3 components of metabolic syndrome for both stone formers and comparators. Censoring time was defined as time from presentation to metabolic stone clinic to last CHIE entry or death. We tested the proportional hazards assumptions by calculating Schoenfield residuals and performing a log-rank test.

Subanalyses for 0 and 1 or 2 previous components, as well as stone type. The main outcome measure was adjusted for number of previous components. Chi-squared test was used to compare prior to year 2000 vs. 2000 onwards for components of MetS.

2.5. Sample Size Calculation

Sample size was calculated estimating a 10% difference (30:40%) in rates of MetS diagnosis between the two groups. Power was set at 80% and significance at 0.05. Sample size was therefore calculated at $n = 172$ per group. Larger numbers have been included to increase power for subanalyses. The 3:1 ratio of controls to cases was used to increase robustness and power.

2.6. Ethical Approval

Ethical approval for this study was granted by the NHS Bristol Research Ethics Committee (Research ethics committee reference: 18/SW/0185; IRAS ID: 240061).

3. Results

3.1. Demographics

There were 828 stone formers and 2484 stone free comparators, with no differences in age or sex between the groups. Stone formers underwent a median 19 years (IQR: 15–22) of follow-up from initial presentation to biochemical clinic. Non-stone formers had data available for the same time period (median 19 years, IQR: 15–22).

There were 361 (43.6%) stone formers who developed metabolic syndrome (MetS), whilst 617 (24.8%) of the stone free comparators developed MetS. Numbers of components and primary stone composition are detailed in Table 2. Deaths were similarly proportioned in the two groups with 113 (13.6%) amongst stone formers, and 366 (14.7%) amongst the comparators.

There were 719 (86.8%) and 2118 (85.3%) stone free comparators without any prior components of MetS. There were 111 (13.4%) and 332 (13.4%) stone free comparators with 1 or 2 components.

Table 2. Demographics of stone formers and stone-free comparators.

		Controls	Stone Formers	HR (95% CI)	p
Age at Presentation (Years), Mean ± SD		49 ± 14	49 ± 14		
Sex, n (%)	Female	723 (29.1%)	241 (29.1%)		
	Male	1761 (70.9%)	587 (70.9%)		
Follow-Up (Years), Median (IQR)		22 (17–27)	22 (17–27)		
Metabolic Syndrome, n (%)		617 (24.8%)	361 (43.6%)	1.77 (1.55–2.03)	<0.001
Metabolic Syndrome Components Developed, n (%)	0	478 (19.2%)	114 (13.8%)		
	1	793 (31.9%)	146 (17.6%)		
	2	596 (24.0%)	172 (20.8%)		
	3	399 (16.1%)	170 (20.5%)		
	4	182 (7.3%)	134 (16.2%)		
	5	36 (1.4%)	83 (1.0%)		
Primary Stone Composition, n (%)	Ca Ox	-	425 (51.3%)	1.82 (1.53–2.16)	<0.001
	Urate	-	21 (2.5%)	3.87 (2.23–6.72)	<0.001
	Ca Po	-	17 (2.1%)	0.89 (0.33–2.38)	0.82
	Struvite	-	5 (0.6%)	0.78 (0.11–5.54)	0.80
	Unclear	-	360 (43.5%)	1.71 (1.43–2.05)	<0.001

3.2. Risk of Metabolic Syndrome in Stone Formers

Stone formers were at significantly increased risk of developing MetS (HR: 1.77; 95% CI: 1.55–2.03, $p < 0.001$) (see Figure 2 and Table 2). This effect was robust to adjustment for presence of previous components (HR: 1.91; 95% CI: 1.66–2.19, $p < 0.001$). This effect was consistent with subanalyses of no previous components (HR: 1.98; 95% CI: 1.69–2.31, $p < 0.001$) and 1 or 2 previous components (HR: 1.54; 95% CI: 1.11–2.14, $p = 0.011$).

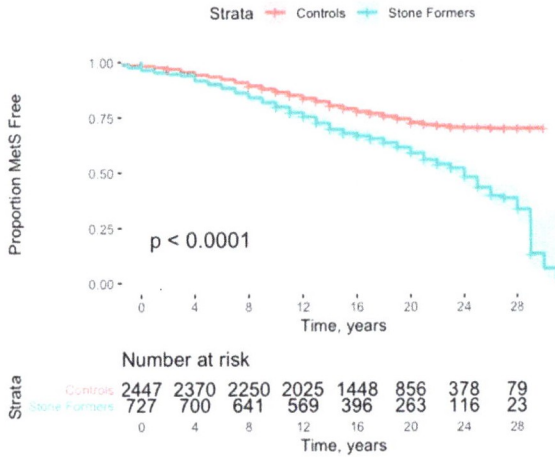

Figure 2. Kaplan Meier curve with 95% CI (confidence interval) for time to development of metabolic syndrome.

Subanalysis of stone type demonstrated significantly higher risk for stone patients compared to their matched comparators presenting with calcium oxalate (HR: 1.82; 95% CI: 1.53–2.16, $p < 0.001$) and urate stones (HR: 3.87; 95% CI: 2.23–6.72, $p < 0.001$) (see Table 1). Other stone types did not carry significant risk of developing MetS.

Subanalysis of individual components of the metabolic syndrome demonstrated SFs were significantly more likely to develop all bar impaired glucose tolerance on both unadjusted and adjusted analyses (see Table 3). Those with the component pre-existing were excluded.

Table 3. Individual components of metabolic syndrome and overall risk. Adjusted for age and sex.

Component	Unadjusted		Adjusted	
	HR (95% CI)	p	HR (95% CI)	p
Impaired Glucose Tolerance	1.19 (0.97–1.46)	0.09	1.17 (0.95–1.43)	0.13
Hypertension	1.56 (1.41–1.81)	<0.001	1.51 (1.33–1.71)	<0.001
BMI > 25	1.41 (1.03–1.26)	0.01	1.11 (1.01–1.24)	0.04
TGL > 1.70	1.58 (1.37–1.83)	<0.001	1.50 (1.30–1.74)	<0.001
HDL < 1.04 for women; <1.29 for men	1.26 (1.09–1.45)	<0.001	1.25 (1.09–1.44)	0.002
Metabolic Syndrome	1.78 (1.56–2.03)	<0.001	1.77 (1.55–2.03)	<0.001

Numbers of patients at follow-up times were as follows: 5-years (control, $n = 2484$; SF, $n = 828$), 10-years (control, $n = 2481$; SF, $n = 827$), 15-years (control, $n = 1938$; SF, $n = 646$), 20-years (control, $n = 1119$; SF, $n = 373$), 25-years (control, $n = 366$; SF, $n = 122$).

There were significantly more patients with previous components of the metabolic syndrome after 2000 than prior (Chi-square, $p < 0.001$), despite this analysis of only those presenting after 2000 still had a significantly increased risk of developing MetS (HR: 2.42, 95% CI: 2.01–2.92, $p < 0.001$). Log rank demonstrated a significant result ($p < 0.001$). Visual inspection of the Schoenfeld residuals did not demonstrate variation around 0, although it did demonstrate a significant result (global Schoenfeld test, $p < 0.001$) (see Figure 3).

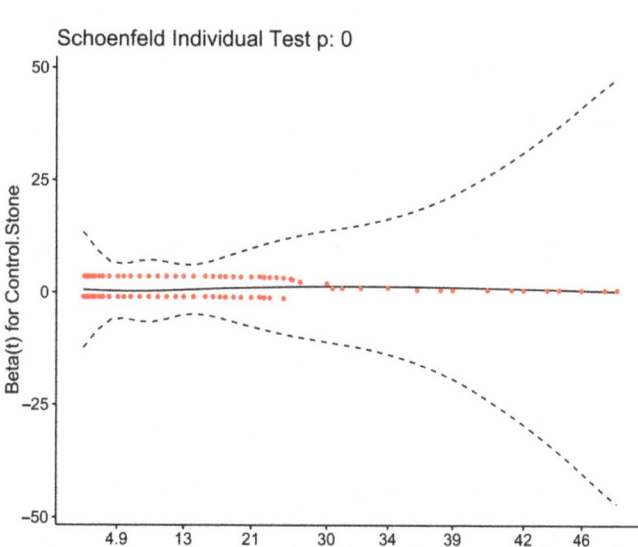

Figure 3. Schoenfeld residuals plotted against time. Loess line with 95% CI.

4. Discussion

This is the first study to examine the risk of metabolic syndrome in stone formers. There was a significant risk (nearly twice as likely) of developing metabolic syndrome in this population, which was more common still in those with uric acid stones.

The main strength of this study is an appropriately powered, significant primary outcome, which is robust to adjustment for previous components. The use of 3:1 matching of study participants to comparators for age and sex, improves power and robustness. Broadly, the sensitivity analyses (log-rank, Schoenfeld residuals and subanalyses) demonstrate results in keeping with the primary outcome.

The major limitation of this study is the risk of under-ascertainment of MetS at baseline (there were only 20 stone formers with MetS), this is reflected in significantly lower MetS components prior to 2000 in both groups. Routine screening of metabolic syndrome components by General Practitioners was not established until after the millennium, which would account for the previously mentioned observation. One would expect a higher number of stone formers to have pre-existing MetS, given that they are more likely to develop KSD [3]. However, the risk of under-ascertainment is likely to be inherent to both groups. We have also adjusted for prior components for both groups, and performed subanalyses on development of MetS with 0, 1, and 2 previous components. All of these analyses demonstrate highly significant results, increasing the likelihood that stone formers are indeed at increased risk of MetS.

There are several other weaknesses to this study. Firstly, the dataset used, Care and Health Information Exchange (CHIE) uses data inputted by general practitioners. Primary care data are known to be more variable and less accurate than secondary care data [17]. It was also not possible to match patient's address' and GP practice's and therefore we were unable to adjust for deprivation. However, the expected results are significant (i.e., urate stones increase risk of MetS and increased risk of recurrence in stone formers with MetS), and therefore there is no risk of type 2 error. Secondly, risk of type 1 error may be present given the multiple testing in the secondary outcomes, and larger studies are needed to corroborate these findings. Lastly, there may be an argument that stone referrals to a tertiary referral service are not representative of the general stone forming population. However, the recurrence rate is similar to previously documented series (around 40% at 10 years in this cohort) [18], only a small proportion were started on prophylactic medication (16%) and there were similar ratios of stone types to previous series [6,19]. Due to these reasons, we believe this dataset is representative.

The increased risk of MetS in the stone forming population is significant given the rising prevalence of kidney stone disease (KSD), which was 10% in 2015–2016 in USA [2]. This translates into 38.2 million Americans who have had a kidney stone and are therefore at roughly twice the risk of developing MetS, with the associated 2- to 4-fold increased risk in cardiovascular disease [15]. It is should be noted it is unlikely to be all stone formers who develop MetS as there are alternative causes of KSD (genetic, infection, drugs, etc.) that have no association with MetS or cardiovascular disease [20].

It is clear that insulin resistance and renal lipotoxicity are the main drivers of stone formation in the MetS population [11,21]. However, it is not clear why stone formers are at increased risk of developing MetS. Our observation that stone formers are more likely to develop MetS correlates with previous studies on the increased risk of developing diabetes [13] and hypertension [14] in stone formers. Both MetS and DM are characterized by insulin resistance, which leads to urinary acidification and increased uric acid excretion [6,22] with a resulting higher proportion of uric acid stones [23]. Hypertension is also associated with urinary acidification along with hypocitraturia [24], both risk factors for stone formation. However, there is no evidence that kidney stones, or abnormalities in 24 h urinary biochemistry influence the development of MetS or its components.

Intriguingly, the link between KSD and MetS is reflected in the genetics literature. In genome wide association studies, two single nucleotide polymorphisms (rs780093 and rs1260326) within a single gene (*GCKR*) are associated with both KSD [25,26] and MetS [27]. This gene encodes glucokinase regulator protein, which is mainly expressed in the liver [28]. Although not yet demonstrated in functional studies, clinically these variants are associated with higher triglycerides and higher fasting plasma glucose [29], both of which are components of MetS and risk factors for KSD. KSD is therefore likely to be a result of metabolic derangements, given the association with these variants (no renal expression of *GCKR*) and the associated risk of KSD with higher triglycerides, higher fasting plasma glucose and MetS.

If KSD is indeed a symptom of an underlying metabolic derangement, rather than vice versa, then there may be evidence of metabolic dysfunction at presentation. It is unclear in the literature whether there is evidence of insulin resistance or renal lipotoxicity, or its surrogates (dyslipidaemia or high BMI) at this point, and we have discussed the risk of under-ascertainment of MetS components earlier. Interestingly, Sagesaka et al. demonstrated that type 2 diabetes could be predicted up to 10 years before the patient developed the condition using the same factors used to diagnose metabolic syndrome [30]. Unfortunately, they did not examine if the components of MetS rose and fell, respectively, as fasting plasma glucose did.

Futures studies should examine the presence of metabolic syndrome components in stone formers prospectively, examining risk of recurrence with metabolic syndrome and development of metabolic syndrome. The involvement of geno- and phenotype correlations should be considered. Preventative measures for both recurrent stones and components of metabolic syndrome should be trialled. More work also needs to be done on primary prevention and effect on patients quality of life [31,32].

Routine assessment for components of MetS should be standard when assessing a stone formers given the further risk of KSD and, perhaps more importantly, the long-term cardiovascular implications [15].

5. Conclusions

Kidney stone formers are at increased risk of developing metabolic syndrome, which is commoner with uric acid stones. A stone is likely a 'symptom' of an underlying, perhaps covert, metabolic derangement in idiopathic stone formers given the described pathophysiology.

This increased risk has both individual and health policy implications given the associated cardiovascular outcomes. Assessment for metabolic syndrome should be standard for patients presenting with kidney stones.

Author Contributions: Study design/concept: R.M.G., B.S.; Data collection: R.M.G.; Data analysis: R.M.G.; Manuscript draft: R.M.G.; Critical appraisal of manuscript: R.M.G., P.C., P.R., B.S. All authors have read and agreed to the published version of the manuscript.

Funding: Robert Geraghty is a National Institute for Health Research funded Academic Clinical Fellow.

Institutional Review Board Statement: Ethical approval for this study was granted by the NHS Bristol Research Ethics Committee (Research ethics committee reference: 18/SW/0185; IRAS ID: 240061).

Informed Consent Statement: Patient consent was waived as this is a retrospective cohort study. Ethical approval was sought and gained to not gain patients consent to access their records. Ethical approval was granted on the provision that only the authors (who are all involved in these patient's care) had access to the data.

Data Availability Statement: As data is identifiable it will not be made available as per ethical approval.

Acknowledgments: We would like to thank the Care and Health Information Analytics team for providing the comparator data. We would like to acknowledge Valerie Walker for initiating the Southampton stone database.

Conflicts of Interest: The authors declare no conflict of interest.

Appendix A

Read codes for Kidney stone disease used to exclude patients:
a. Readcode version 2 '4G4' and below within hierarchy.
b. CTV3

'XE0dk'	—	Kidney stone
'K1200'	—	Staghorn calculus
'X30Po'	—	Calyceal renal calculus
'X30Pp'	—	Calculus in calyceal diverticulum
'X30Pq'	—	Calculus in renal pelvis
'X30Pr'	—	Calculus in pelviureteric junction
'XM14o'	—	Uric acid renal calculus
'K120z'	—	Renal calculus NOS

References

1. Geraghty, R.M.; Cook, P.; Walker, V.; Somani, B.K. Evaluation of the economic burden of kidney stone disease in the UK: A retro-spective cohort study with a mean follow-up of 19 years. *BJU Int.* **2020**, *125*, 586–594. [CrossRef]
2. Chewcharat, A.; Curhan, G. Trends in the prevalence of kidney stones in the United States from 2007 to 2016. *Urolithiasis* **2021**, *49*, 27–39. [CrossRef]
3. Geraghty, R.; Abdi, A.; Somani, B.; Cook, P.; Roderick, P. Does chronic hyperglycaemia increase the risk of kidney stone disease? results from a systematic review and meta-analysis. *BMJ Open* **2020**, *10*, e032094. [CrossRef] [PubMed]
4. Einhorn, D.; Reaven, G.M.; Cobin, R.H.; Ford, E.; Ganda, O.P.; Handelsman, Y.; Hellman, R.; Jellinger, P.S.; Kendall, D.; Krauss, R.M.; et al. American College of Endocrinology position statement on the insulin resistance syndrome. *Endocr. Pract.* **2003**, *9*, 237–252. [CrossRef]
5. Abate, N.; Chandalia, M.; Cabo-Chan, A.V.; Moe, O.W.; Sakhaee, K. The metabolic syndrome and uric acid nephrolithiasis: Novel features of renal manifestation of insulin resistance. *Kidney Int.* **2004**, *65*, 386–392. [CrossRef] [PubMed]

6. Kadlec, A.O.; Greco, K.; Fridirici, Z.C.; Hart, S.T.; Vellos, T.; Turk, T.M. Metabolic Syndrome and Urinary Stone Composition: What Factors Matter Most? *Urology* **2012**, *80*, 805–810. [CrossRef]
7. Moore, J.X.; Chaudhary, N.; Akinyemiju, T. Metabolic Syndrome Prevalence by Race/Ethnicity and Sex in the United States, National Health and Nutrition Examination Survey, 1988–2012. *Prev. Chronic Dis.* **2017**, *14*, E24. [CrossRef] [PubMed]
8. Taylor, E.N.; Stampfer, M.J.; Curhan, G.C. Obesity, weight gain, and the risk of kidney stones. *JAMA* **2005**, *293*, 455–462. [CrossRef]
9. Madore, F.; Stampfer, M.J.; Rimm, E.B.; Curhan, G.C. Nephrolithiasis and Risk of Hypertension. *Am. J. Hypertens.* **1998**, *11*, 46–53. [CrossRef]
10. Akoudad, S.; Szklo, M.; McAdams, M.A.; Fulop, T.; Anderson, C.A.; Coresh, J.; Köttgen, A. Correlates of kidney stone disease differ by race in a multi-ethnic middle-aged population: The ARIC study. *Prev. Med.* **2010**, *51*, 416–420. [CrossRef] [PubMed]
11. Torricelli, F.C.M.; De, S.K.; Gebreselassie, S.; Li, I.; Sarkissian, C.; Monga, M. Urolithiasis/Endourology Dyslipidemia and Kidney Stone Risk. *J. Urol.* **2014**, *191*, 667–672. [CrossRef] [PubMed]
12. Weinberg, J. Lipotoxicity. *Kidney Int.* **2006**, *70*, 1560–1566. [CrossRef]
13. Chung, S.-D.; Chen, Y.-K.; Lin, H.-C. Increased Risk of Diabetes in Patients with Urinary Calculi: A 5-Year Followup Study. *J. Urol.* **2011**, *186*, 1888–1893. [CrossRef] [PubMed]
14. Kittanamongkolchai, W.; Mara, K.C.; Mehta, R.A.; Vaughan, L.E.; Denic, A.; Knoedler, J.J.; Enders, F.T.; Lieske, J.C.; Rule, A.D. Risk of Hypertension among First-Time Symptomatic Kidney Stone Formers. *Clin. J. Am. Soc. Nephrol.* **2017**, *12*, 476–482. [CrossRef] [PubMed]
15. Bonora, E. The metabolic syndrome and cardiovascular disease. *Ann. Med.* **2006**, *38*, 64–80. [CrossRef]
16. Walker, V.; Stansbridge, E.M.; Griffin, D.G. Demography and biochemistry of 2800 patients from a renal stones clinic. *Ann. Clin. Biochem. Int. J. Lab. Med.* **2013**, *50*, 127–139. [CrossRef]
17. Thiru, K.; Hassey, A.; Sullivan, F. Systematic review of scope and quality of electronic patient record data in primary care. *BMJ* **2003**, *326*, 1070. [CrossRef]
18. Ljunghall, S.; Danielson, B.G. A Prospective Study of Renal Stone Recurrences. *Br. J. Urol.* **1984**, *56*, 122–124. [CrossRef]
19. Daudon, M.; Lacour, B.; Jungers, P. Influence of body size on urinary stone composition in men and women. *Urol. Res.* **2006**, *34*, 193–199. [CrossRef]
20. Halbritter, J.; Baum, M.; Hynes, A.M.; Rice, S.J.; Thwaites, D.T.; Gucev, Z.S.; Fisher, B.; Spaneas, L.; Porath, J.D.; Braun, D.A.; et al. Fourteen Monogenic Genes Account for 15% of Nephrolithiasis/Nephrocalcinosis. *J. Am. Soc. Nephrol.* **2014**, *26*, 543–551. [CrossRef]
21. Bobulescu, I.A.; Dubree, M.; Zhang, J.; McLeroy, P.; Moe, O.W. Effect of renal lipid accumulation on proximal tubule Na^+/H^+ exchange and am-monium secretion. *Am. J. Physiol. Ren. Physiol.* **2008**, *294*, F1315–F1322. [CrossRef]
22. Maalouf, N.M.; Cameron, M.A.; Moe, O.W.; Sakhaee, K. Metabolic Basis for Low Urine pH in Type 2 Diabetes. *Clin. J. Am. Soc. Nephrol.* **2010**, *5*, 1277–1281. [CrossRef] [PubMed]
23. Wiederkehr, M.R.; Moe, O.W. Uric Acid Nephrolithiasis: A Systemic Metabolic Disorder. *Clin. Rev. Bone Miner. Metab.* **2011**, *9*, 207–217. [CrossRef] [PubMed]
24. Hartman, C.; Friedlander, J.I.; Moreira, D.M.; Leavitt, D.A.; Hoenig, D.M.; Smith, A.D.; Okeke, Z. Does hypertension impact 24-hour urine parameters in patients with nephro-lithiasis? *Urology* **2015**, *85*, 539–543. [CrossRef] [PubMed]
25. Howles, S.A.; Wiberg, A.; Goldsworthy, M.; Bayliss, A.L.; Gluck, A.K.; Ng, M.; Grout, E.; Tanikawa, C.; Kamatani, Y.; Terao, C.; et al. Genetic variants of calcium and vitamin D metabolism in kidney stone disease. *Nat. Commun.* **2019**, *10*, 5175. [CrossRef] [PubMed]
26. Tanikawa, C.; Kamatani, Y.; Terao, C.; Usami, M.; Takahashi, A.; Momozawa, Y.; Suzuki, K.; Ogishima, S.; Shimizu, A.; Satoh, M.; et al. Novel Risk Loci Identified in a Genome-Wide Association Study of Urolithiasis in a Japanese Population. *J. Am. Soc. Nephrol.* **2019**, *30*, 855–864. [CrossRef]
27. Oh, S.-W.; Lee, J.-E.; Shin, E.; Kwon, H.; Choe, E.K.; Choi, S.-Y.; Rhee, H.; Choi, S.H. Genome-wide association study of metabolic syndrome in Korean populations. *PLoS ONE* **2020**, *15*, e0227357. [CrossRef]
28. Jiang, L.; Wang, M.; Lin, S.; Jian, R.; Li, X.; Chan, J.; Dong, G.; Fang, H.; Robinson, A.E.; Snyder, M.P.; et al. A Quantitative Proteome Map of the Human Body. *Cell* **2020**, *183*, 269–283. [CrossRef]
29. Vaxillaire, M.; Cavalcanti-Proença, C.; Dechaume, A.; Tichet, J.; Marre, M.; Balkau, B.; Froguel, P. For the DESIR study group The Common P446L Polymorphism in GCKR Inversely Modulates Fasting Glucose and Triglyceride Levels and Reduces Type 2 Diabetes Risk in the DESIR Prospective General French Population. *Diabetes* **2008**, *57*, 2253–2257. [CrossRef]
30. Sagesaka, H.; Sato, Y.; Someya, Y.; Tamura, Y.; Shimodaira, M.; Miyakoshi, T.; Hirabayashi, K.; Koike, H.; Yamashita, K.; Watada, H.; et al. Type 2 Diabetes: When Does It Start? *J. Endocr. Soc.* **2018**, *2*, 476–484. [CrossRef]
31. Gamage, K.N.; Jamnadass, E.; Sulaiman, S.K.; Pietropaolo, A.; Aboumarzouk, O.; Somani, B.K. The role of fluid intake in the prevention of kidney stone disease: A systematic review over the last two decades. *Turk. J. Urol.* **2020**, *46* (Suppl. S1), S92. [CrossRef] [PubMed]
32. New, F.; Somani, B.K. A complete world literature review on quality of life (QOL) in patients with kidney stone disease (KSD). *Curr. Urol. Rep.* **2016**, *17*, 88. [CrossRef] [PubMed]

6.

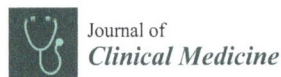

Article

Quality Assessment of CEUS in Individuals with Small Renal Masses—Which Individual Factors Are Associated with High Image Quality?

Paul Spiesecke [1], Thomas Fischer [1], Frank Friedersdorff [2], Bernd Hamm [1] and Markus Herbert Lerchbaumer [1],*

1. Department of Radiology, Charité-Universitätsmedizin Berlin, 10117 Berlin, Germany; paul.spiesecke@charite.de (P.S.); thom.fischer@charite.de (T.F.); bernd.hamm@charite.de (B.H.)
2. Department of Urology, Charité-Universitätsmedizin Berlin, 10117 Berlin, Germany; frank.friedersdorff@charite.de
* Correspondence: markus.lerchbaumer@charite.de; Tel.: +49-(0)-30-450-657084; Fax: +49-(0)-30-450-7557901

Received: 17 November 2020; Accepted: 13 December 2020; Published: 17 December 2020

Abstract: Obesity and bowel gas are known to impair image quality in abdominal ultrasound (US). The present study aims at identifying individual factors in B-mode US that influence contrast-enhanced US (CEUS) image quality to optimize further imaging workup of incidentally detected focal renal masses. We retrospectively analyzed renal CEUS of focal renal masses ≤ 4 cm performed at our center in 143 patients between 2016 and 2020. Patient and lesion characteristics were tested for their influence on focal and overall image quality assessed by two experienced radiologists using Likert scales. Effects of significant variables were quantified by receiver operating characteristics (ROC) curve analysis with area under the curve (AUC), and combined effects were assessed by binary logistic regression. Shrunken kidney, kidney depth, lesion depth, lesion size, and exophytic lesion growth were found to influence focal renal lesion image quality, and all factors except lesion size also influenced overall image quality. Combination of all parameters except kidney depth best predicted good CEUS image quality showing an AUC of 0.91 ($p < 0.001$, 95%-CI 0.863–0.958). The B-mode US parameters investigated can identify patients expected to have good CEUS image quality and thus help select the most suitable contrast-enhanced imaging strategy for workup of renal lesions.

Keywords: CEUS; contrast-enhanced ultrasound; renal ultrasound; image quality; small renal mass (3–5)

---

1. Introduction

Renal lesions are estimated to occur in 13% to 27% of the general population [1–3]. Small renal masses (SRMs) defined as lesions ≤ 4 cm, tend to be asymptomatic and are often detected incidentally on imaging [4,5]. It is generally known that the incidence of malignancy increases with the size of a SRM [6]. Therefore, early and accurate diagnosis of small renal lesions is very important to plan further patient management and ensure good patient outcome.

Since the risk of malignancy in solid renal tumors is high with incidences of 87.2% and 83.9% reported by Frank et al. and Kutikov et al., respectively [7,8], the choice of a suitable imaging method for reliable differentiation of malignant from benign lesions is essential for the diagnostic process. Often, a renal tumor is detected as an incidental finding in a routine ultrasound (US) examination, and the question as to the most appropriate further imaging strategy arises. Although US has many advantages including the absence of ionizing radiation as well as low costs and high availability, a systematic review by Vogel et al. identified poor diagnostic performance of conventional US in renal tumors [9], making contrast-enhanced imaging necessary for a reliable characterization. In this review, Vogel et al. showed comparable sensitivity for contrast-enhanced computed tomography (ceCT), contrast-enhanced magnetic resonance imaging (ceMRI) and contrast-enhanced ultrasound (CEUS) [9]. Furthermore, CEUS turned out to have higher diagnostic accuracy than ceCT in the evaluation of complex cystic renal masses [9].

Besides diagnostic accuracy, the setting of a contrast-enhanced examination plays a decisive role: while ceCT still remains the first-line imaging modality for SRMs, MRI has become more widely used over the last decade and also avoids radiation exposure, but its general use is limited by its availability and cost [10]. On the other hand, CEUS is superior regarding the evaluation of microcirculation as it uses a strictly intravascular contrast agent consisting of gas-filled microbubbles [10].

For CEUS of focal liver lesions, it has been shown that diagnostic confidence is improved by good examination conditions [11]. The authors of this study defined difficult ultrasound (US) conditions as the presence of meteorism, distinct steatosis, liver cirrhosis with inhomogeneous tissue, and obesity with a body mass index (BMI) > 30 kg/m^2 [11].

In 2018, Sidhu et al. published the EFSUMB (European Federation of Societies for Ultrasound in Medicine and Biology) guidelines and recommendations for the use of CEUS in non-hepatic applications [12]. Next to renal ischemia, they identify focal renal lesions as the main indication for CEUS in the kidney. The focal renal lesions that can be diagnosed using CEUS are pseudotumors, cystic, indeterminate and solid masses as well as renal infections [12]. Thus, indications for CEUS include the whole range of SRMs investigated here, and the question arises of which patient-related imaging factors must be met to allow a CEUS examination likely to yield sufficient image quality for correct diagnostic characterization. This should help in deciding, in each case, whether a patient would benefit more from CEUS or cross-sectional imaging after initial sonographic detection of a SRM.

To our knowledge, this is the first study systematically analyzing essential patient and lesion characteristics and their influence on CEUS image quality in renal US.

2. Materials and Methods

This retrospective study was registered with our institution's ethics committee (EA1/320/20). The oral and written informed consent of all patients was obtained before the examination. All study data were collected in compliance with the principles expressed in the 2002 Declaration of Helsinki.

2.1. Study Population

A database query for CEUS examinations of focal renal lesions performed in our hospital's interdisciplinary ultrasound center between January 2016 and May 2020 was conducted. The cases retrieved by this search were screened regarding the following inclusion criteria: (I) age ≥ 18 years, (II) CEUS examination of a focal renal lesion ≤ 4 cm, and (III) sufficient image data for quality assessment (stored cine loops and multiple images). Exclusion criteria were (I) autosomal-dominant polycystic kidney disease and (II) no lesion or other indication for CEUS (assessment of renal perfusion).

2.2. CEUS Examination

Gray-scale B-mode US of the kidney was performed for lesion detection and for assessment of kidney size, echogenicity, and homogeneity using high-end ultrasound systems with a 1–6 MHz convex array transducer (Aplio i500/i900, Canon Medical Systems Corporation, Tochigi, Japan; Acuson Sequoia, Siemens Healthineers, Erlangen, Germany). The kidney was routinely examined in modified longitudinal and transverse planes and, if necessary, in deep inspiration and with optimized scanning positions.

CEUS examinations were performed during clinical routine using high-end ultrasound systems with up-to-date CEUS-specific protocols available at the time of the examination. The examinations were performed at 1–6 MHz with convex array transducers. A bolus of 1.6 mL of ultrasound contrast agent (SonoVue®, Bracco Imaging, Milan, Italy) was administered in all patients, and a very low mechanical index (MI < 0.1) was used to avoid early microbubble destruction. Penetration depth on CEUS was adapted by the investigator to clearly identify the target lesion and whole kidney.

Baseline B-mode US and CEUS (for qualitative assessment of contrast enhancement pattern) were performed by a single highly experienced radiologist with more than ten years of experience in CEUS (EFSUMB level 3).

The associated data concerning the included patients were reviewed to collect individual information. The Radiology Information System (RIS) was used to cover age and gender.

2.3. Assessment of Image Quality

Image quality was evaluated by two radiologists in consensus, one of them an EFSUMB level 3 examiner and both experienced in the field of renal CEUS. One factor assessed was presence of reduced parenchymal thickness or shrunken kidney (renal atrophy). Kidney depth and lesion depth were determined as the shortest distance of the renal capsule/superficial part of the lesion to the probe. Cases were stratified by lesion size and localization in the left versus right kidney and site within the kidney—upper third, middle or lower third—on representative CEUS loops, if not described in the diagnostic reports. Image quality at the target site (lesion) and overall image quality (kidney) were assessed in terms of diagnostic confidence by two experienced readers using an ordinal scoring system (Likert scale): 1—insufficient quality, 2—poor quality, 3—adequate quality, 4—good quality, 5—excellent quality. Representative examples of CEUS images illustrating different image qualities are shown in Figure 1.

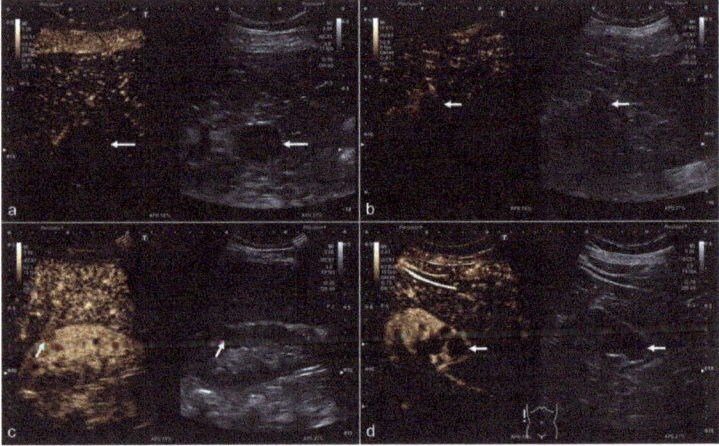

Figure 1. Examples of images illustrating different image quality scores. Images illustrating image quality of four different contrast-enhanced ultrasound (CEUS) examinations performed with the same US system, convex probe, and standardized imaging protocol (gain, dynamic range) with bolus injection of 1.6 mL SonoVue (Bracco Imaging): (**a**,**b**) Low image quality of a cystic and solid renal lesion, score of 1 for focal image quality in case of (**a**) and score of 2 for (**b**). (**c**,**d**) High image quality of a small solid lesion with a size of 12 mm (**c**) and an exophytic lesion at the lower pole of the kidney (**d**), both assigned scores of 5 for focal lesion.

2.4. Statistical Analysis

Continuous variables are reported as median and interquartile range (IQR) and categorical variables as absolute/total numbers (n/N) and percentages in brackets. The aim of our analysis is to identify patient and lesion factors that affect CEUS image quality. Therefore, image quality scores—ordinally scaled—were correlated with the presence of various patient- and lesion-related variables using the Chi^2 test for variables measured in ratio scale and the Kruskal-Wallis test for ordinally scaled variables. Effects were analyzed for both focal (site of renal lesion) and overall image quality. In addition, a univariate ANOVA was performed to detect possible uncertainties. Moreover, post hoc testing with Bonferroni correction was done to ensure that at least two image quality groups differed statistically significantly from each other. To investigate the interdependence of impact of lesion location (right vs. left kidney and kidney third) on image quality, a two-factorial ANOVA of these two factors was performed.

For the parameters identified to have a statistically significant influence on image quality, the effect was quantified by receiver operating characteristics (ROC) curve analysis with quantification of the area under the curve (AUC). Therefore, good image quality was defined as a score of 4 or 5 on the Likert scale as described above. Furthermore, different combinations of individual parameters with a statistically significant influence on image quality were tested by binary logistic regression to determine the AUCs quantifying the influence of the combined parameters. The best combination of individual parameters was identified as the combination with the largest AUC and the smallest number of included parameters compared to other combinations with the same AUC.

A two-sided significance level of $\alpha = 0.05$ was considered appropriate to indicate statistical significance. All statistical analyses were performed using the SPSS software (IBM Corp. Released 2019. IBM SPSS Statistics for Windows, Version 26.0. IBM Corp: Armonk, NY, USA).

3. Results

3.1. Study Population

The final study population included 143 patients with at least one renal target lesion ≤ 4 cm and sufficient stored image data for quality assessment. The patients' baseline characteristics are presented in Table 1. Ninety-four of the initially identified CEUS examinations were excluded since they were repeat follow-up examinations of already included patients. The study patients had a median age of 62 years (IQR, 52–75 years). Cystic renal lesions were found in 78.3% of the cases and 21.7% as solid renal lesions. Overall mean lesion depth was 61 mm (IQR, 46–74 mm).

Table 1. Baseline characteristics of included patients.

Variable	Value
Characteristics of the patients	
Age [years]	62 (52–75)
Female sex	43/143 (30.1%)
Characteristics of the kidney	
Kidney depth [mm]	48 (39–62)
Shrunken kidney	37/143 (25.9%)
Reduced cortical thickness	40/143 (28.0%)
Characteristics of the lesion	
Cystic	112/143 (78.3%)
Solid	31/143 (21.7%)
Depth of renal lesion [mm]	61 (46–74)
Largest lesion diameter [mm]	20 (14–26)
Left side	72/143 (50.3%)
Right side	71/143 (49.7%)
Upper third	45/143 (31.5%)
Middle third	65/143 (45.5%)
Lower third	33/143 (23.1%)
Exophytic lesion growth	60/143 (42.0%)

Abbreviations: IQR denotes interquartile range.

Presented are the baseline characteristics of the study population subdivided into patient- and lesion-related features. Continuous variables are given as median (IQR), categorical variables as absolute/total numbers (n/N) and percentages in brackets.

3.2. Assessment of Image Quality

Arithmetic means of image quality scores were 3.7 and 3.6 for focal and overall image quality, respectively. Focal image quality scores 1–5 were distributed as follows: 4 (2.8%), 15 (10.5%), 43 (30.1%), 42 (29.4%), and 39 (27.3%). For overall image quality, score distribution was: 6 (4.2%), 22 (15.4%), 39 (27.3%), 28 (19.6%), and 48 (33.6%). Correlation with individual patient and lesion characteristics yielded the following results: there were no strong correlations between imaging quality and age, sex, reduced cortical thickness or entity, localization, and size of lesion (Table 2). A statistically significant increase in image quality was found for (I) exophytic growth of focal renal lesion, (II) absence of shrunken kidneys, (III) lower lesion depth, and (IV) lower depth of lesion-bearing kidney (Table 2, Figure 2). For intrarenal lesion site (upper, middle, lower third), the Chi^2 test yielded no correlation with image quality ($p = 0.064$), whereas ANOVA reached significance ($p = 0.040$). With the restrictive approach used here, we do not interpret the results as showing a strong correlation in order to satisfy the discrepancy between the two applied statistical tests.

Table 2. Influence of patient and lesion characteristics on focal and overall image quality.

Variable	Focal Quality		Overall Quality	
	Nonparametric test	ANOVA	Nonparametric test	ANOVA
Age	0.750 [2]	0.809	0.387 [2]	0.460
Sex	0.290 [1]	0.296	0.426 [1]	0.434
Entity [3]	0.433 [1]	0.441	0.134 [1]	0.135
Reduced parenchymal thickness	0.807 [1]	0.814	0.275 [1]	0.280
Shrunken kidney	<0.001 [1]	<0.001	<0.001 [1]	<0.001
Kidney depth	<0.001 [2]	<0.001	<0.001 [2]	<0.001
Lesion depth	<0.001 [2]	<0.001	<0.001 [2]	<0.001
Lesion size	0.006 [2]	0.004	0.385 [2]	0.494
Exophytic lesion growth	0.043 [1]	0.042	0.021 [1]	0.020
Side	0.321 [1]	0.328	0.923 [1]	0.926
Intrarenal third	0.064 [1]	0.040	0.156 [1]	0.211

[1] tested with the Chi^2 test, [2] tested with Kruskal-Wallis test; [3] entity was stratified as cystic versus solid lesion; ANOVA denotes analysis of variance.

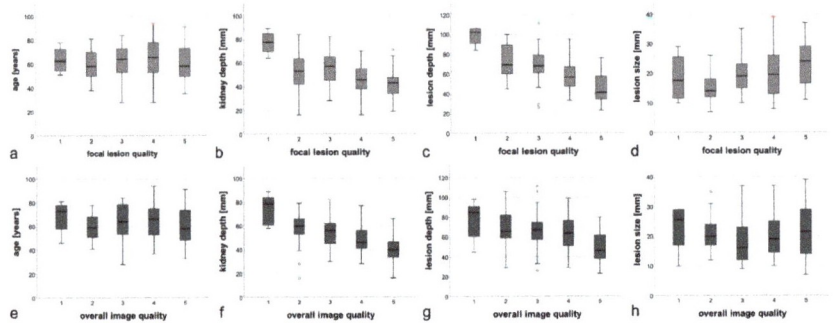

Figure 2. Distribution of continuous variables age, kidney depth, lesion depth and lesion size in focal and overall image quality classes. Boxplots of the distributions of the continuous variables across the five image quality classes (Likert scores) for focal image quality (**a**–**d**) and overall image quality (**e**–**h**). The results of the statistical tests are outlined in Table 2. (**a**,**e**) The age of the patient showed, neither for focal nor for overall image quality, a statistically significant relationship which could be visualized using boxplots.(**b**,**f**) The kidney depth showed for focal image quality, as well as overall image quality lower mean kidney depth for higher image quality.(**c**,**g**) The same relationship as described for kidney depth (**b**,**f**) applies for lesion depth and image quality. (**d**,**h**) The lesion size shows higher mean lesion size for higher focal image quality. For overall image quality, no tendency is visible.

Table 2 presents the results of the statistical tests investigating effects on focal and overall image quality. For each variable and both focal and overall image quality, a nonparametric test and an ANOVA were performed to account for possible uncertainties.

The two-sided ANOVA confirmed the results given in Table 2, showing both focal lesion quality ($p = 0.155$) and overall quality ($p = 0.127$) not to be impacted by the combined lesion location parameters (right/left kidney and intrarenal lesion site).

3.3. Post Hoc Tests

The results of post hoc ANOVA confirmed that sex, age, lesion type, shrunken kidney, and side of involved kidney had no statistically significant impact on focal or overall image quality. Additionally, intrarenal lesion localization (third) was shown to have no statistically significant effect on focal or overall image quality, whereas univariate ANOVA of focal lesion quality identified an effect of intrarenal lesion localization ($p = 0.046$), which was confirmed by the Chi^2 test ($p = 0.064$). As expected from univariate ANOVA, testing with Bonferroni correction also identified no statistically significant effect of lesion size on overall image quality.

For both focal and overall image quality, statistically significant ($p \leq 0.05$) differences between at least two groups were found in groupwise comparisons of image quality performed with Bonferroni correction for the following parameters: shrunken kidney, kidney depth, lesion depth, and exophytic lesion growth. For lesion size, a statistically significant difference between at least two groups was found only for the effect on focal image quality.

3.4. ROC Analysis

ROC analysis was performed to quantify the characteristic's influence on reaching high image quality (≥ 4 Likert scores). The results of ROC curve analysis with the area under the curve (AUC) for continuous and categorial variables are presented in Table 3 and in Figure 3.

Table 3. ROC analysis to quantify effects of variables predicting high image quality.

Variable	Focal Quality			Overall Quality		
	AUC	Asymptotic significance	Asymptotic 95%-CI	AUC	Asymptotic significance	Asymptotic 95%-CI
Shrunken kidney	0.684	<0.001	0.593–0.776	0.748	<0.001	0.664–0.832
Kidney depth	0.744	<0.001	0.661–0.827	0.776	<0.001	0.696–0.856
Lesion depth	0.800	<0.001	0.727–0.873	0.695	<0.001	0.609–0.781
Lesion size	0.625	0.011	0.534–0.715	–	–	–
Exophytic lesion growth	0.614	0.020	0.521–0.707	0.502	0.049	0.406–0.597

ROC denotes receiver operating characteristics, AUC denotes area under the curve, CI denotes confidence interval.

ROC analysis was performed to quantify effects of statistically significant variables influencing image quality (Table 2). The ROC curves of all variables showed statistical significance. Nevertheless, the asymptotic 95%-CI of exophytic lesion growth strikes 0.5 in overall image quality and was therefore not considered in further evaluation.

Presented are receiver operating characteristics (ROC) curves of individual parameters and the best combination, as presented in Table 4, influencing focal image quality (Likert score of 4 as cut-off). Diagonal segments were produced by ties.

AUC revealed lesion depth to be associated with focal image quality and kidney depth to be the strongest predictor of overall image quality, confirming the theoretical expectation regarding image quality assessment.

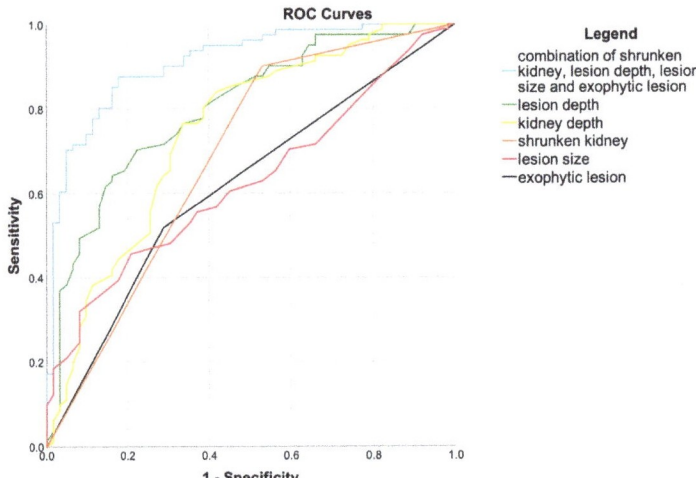

Figure 3. ROC curves of the single parameters and the best combination.

Table 4. ROC analysis of combined variables and their effect in predicting high (score of 4 or 5) focal image quality.

No.	Combined Variables					ROC Analysis		
	Shrunken kidney	Kidney depth	Lesion depth	Lesion size	Exophytic lesion growth	AUC	Asymptotic significance	Asymptotic 95%-CI
1		X	X			0.812	<0.001	0.741–0.883
2	X	X	X			0.863	<0.001	0.805–0.921
3	X				X	0.773	<0.001	0.697–0.850
4			X	X	X	0.843	<0.001	0.777–0.909
5			X	X		0.834	<0.001	0.767–0.902
6	X		X	X		0.893	<0.001	0.841–0.945
7		X	X	X	X	0.851	<0.001	0.787–0.915
8	X	X		X	X	0.870	<0.001	0.812–0.928
9	X		X	X	X	0.910	<0.001	0.863–0.958
10	X	X	X	X	X	0.910	<0.001	0.863–0.957
11		X	X	X		0.842	<0.001	0.777–0.907

Since all variables were quantified regarding effect on high focal image quality (score of 4 or 5), eleven different combinations were investigated. With each of them, a bivariate logistic regression and ROC analysis were performed. Presented are the combinations, with 'X' indicating the single parameters to participate in the bivariate logistic regression and their AUC with asymptotic significance and 95%-CI. Combination No. 9 generates the largest AUC, while including one variable less than combination No. 10. ROC denotes receiver operating characteristics, AUC denotes area under the curve, CI denotes confidence interval.

3.5. Combined ROC Analysis

As described in the Methods section, the combination of shrunken kidney, lesion depth, lesion size, and exophytic lesion growth were identified to be the most suitable combination of parameters (Table 4) showing strong correlation with good focal image quality (score of 4 or 5). with an effect size of an AUC of 0.91 (asymptotic 95%-CI: 0.863–0.958) and asymptotic statistical significance of $p < 0.001$.

4. Discussion

The major results of the present study can be summarized as follows: (I) CEUS image quality is reduced in shrunken kidneys and improved when examining exophytically growing lesions, and with shorter distance of the kidney and the lesion from the transducer; this applies to both focal and overall image quality; (II) focal, but not overall, image quality increases with lesion size, while patient age and sex, lesion entity, reduced parenchymal thickness and lesion localization do not impact CEUS image quality; and (III) the significant parameters just mentioned above improve focal image quality more markedly than the individual parameters alone, with the combination of shrunken kidney, lesion depth, lesion size, and exophytic lesion growth proving to be the most suitable combination.

Putz et al. reported meteorism and obesity as the main patient-related factors with a negative effect on CEUS image quality [11]. While CEUS is predominantly used for liver imaging, renal applications of CEUS have attracted growing interest. Therefore, an interest exists in knowing which patient factors might reliably predict a sufficient CEUS image quality. This is the rationale for our study, which—to our knowledge—is the first systematic analysis of individual patient- and lesion-related factors that have an effect on the image quality of renal CEUS.

Nevertheless, it must be mentioned that not only patient and lesion characteristics influence image quality, and therefore diagnostic accuracy, but also artifacts which are partially CEUS-specific, such as near-field signal loss due to microbubble destruction—which can be influenced by using a specific configuration of the US machine [13,14].

Our results have important implications for the diagnostic workup of SRMs detected on nonenhanced imaging: CEUS shows high diagnostic performance [9] and other advantages including a low rate of side effects [15]. Therefore, CEUS is generally preferred for the characterization of focal renal lesion. A recently published study showed CEUS, even in a small cohort of six pregnant women, to be a safe imaging tool [16]. Knowing beforehand whether a chosen imaging modality is likely to yield a diagnosis can shorten the diagnostic process, improving patient comfort and outcome. Using CEUS only where it is expected to achieve diagnostic quality, its instantaneous diagnosis determines directly if cross-sectional imaging is necessary for cancer staging if a malignant lesion is diagnosed, thus preventing unnecessary imaging in patients with benign lesions.

The prediction as to whether CEUS or MRI might be the better imaging method for further characterization of an SRM incidentally detected by plain B-mode ultrasound also has important economic implications, identifying patients not in need of undergoing MRI.

CEUS benefits—especially shown for renal cysts—from a higher temporal resolution than CT and MRI, allowing real-time evaluation of the enhancement pattern [17–19].

Therefore, immediate workup of an incidental SRM by CEUS in suitable patients can save costs by replacing cross-sectional MRI. Besides, the MRI and CT slots not needed for patients worked up by CEUS can help other patients to obtain their MRI or CT examination more quickly.

Apart from what has been discussed so far, patient preferences should also play a role in selecting an imaging modality. For example, Thorpe et al. found that more than 50% of individuals have a high grade of anxiety during an MRI examination, which could, for instance, promote the occurrence of motion artifacts [20]. Another concern with ceMRI is that gadolinium deposition in the brain has been observed in patients undergoing repeated MRI with administration of a gadolinium-based contrast agent—although its pathologic value is unclear [21,22]. Nevertheless, clinically relevant side effects of iodinated contrast agents used in ceCT are more common: "contrast-induced nephropathy" or "postcontrast acute kidney injury" has an incidence between 5.0% and 6.4% based on meta-analysis data [23–25]. Not being limited by adverse effects such as nephrotoxicity, cumulative radiation exposure or gadolinium deposition, CEUS is well suited for long-term surveillance, for instance, in patients with Bosniak IIF cysts [26].

Besides the image quality expectable in CEUS examination, it must be mentioned that patients with shrunken kidneys might not provide a high image quality, but would suffer from iodinated contrast agents in ceCT, since impaired renal function was found to be associated with contrast-induced nephropathy [24]. Although, as mentioned above, its clinical relevance is subject to controversial discussions, impaired renal function also leads to a reduced elimination of Gadolinium-containing contrast agents used in ceMRI [27]. So an expected low image quality could be relativized by potential harm using the alternative of contrast-enhanced imaging.

Experienced examiners are able to estimate CEUS image quality from B-mode image quality. Nevertheless, our results can help less experienced examiners and allow an objective assessment of expected CEUS image quality in inconclusive cases. Moreover, our approach is straightforward, using criteria that are rapidly assessed such as lesion depth or exophytic lesion growth. Although the two variables show comparable results in our study, lesion depth should be preferred to kidney depth, since this information is also important for lesion characterization rather than for assessing obesity only. Finally, the parameters presented here should be considered together, since the AUC for individual parameters alone are not larger than 0.8 (Table 3). Obviously, an experienced examiner can also characterize SRMs with a lower image quality, but we used high-end US-devices in our study and acquisition of CEUS-loops by an experienced radiologist and vindicate, therefore, our ROC analyses (Tables 3 and 4, Figure 3) with an image quality score of four as cut-off.

4.1. Limitations

Our study is limited by its retrospective and single-center design. Nevertheless, all patients were examined with an identical CEUS protocol. All ultrasound examinations were performed using high-end systems with state-of-the-art CEUS-specific protocols, resulting in generally high image quality. Nevertheless, we compared CEUS loops obtained with a standardized protocol to assess image quality and imaging parameters, and not the image quality of the system as such.

4.2. Conclusions

Focal image quality of CEUS examinations is impaired by shrunken kidney, a large distance of the kidney and lesion from the body surface, and smaller lesion size, while exophytic growth of a focal renal lesion results in better image quality. Awareness of patient and lesion factors that degrade image quality can be used for better patient selection and can thus improve diagnostic confidence of examiners performing CEUS.

Author Contributions: Conceptualization, P.S. and M.H.L.; Formal analysis, P.S., T.F. and M.H.L.; Writing—original draft, P.S. and M.H.L.; Writing—review & editing, P.S., T.F., F.F., B.H. and M.H.L. All authors revised the manuscript critically for important intellectual content and gave final approval of the submitted manuscript. All authors have read and agreed to the published version of the manuscript.

Funding: We acknowledge support from the German Research Foundation (DFG) and the Open Access Publication Fund of Charité-Universitätsmedizin Berlin.

Acknowledgments: The authors thank Bettina Herwig for language editing of the manuscript.

Conflicts of Interest: None of the authors reports a relationship with industry and other relevant entities—financial or otherwise—that might pose a conflict of interest in connection with the submitted article. The following authors report financial activities outside the submitted work: Paul Spiesecke reports no conflict of interest. Thomas Fischer reports having received consultancy honoraria from Bracco and Canon Medical Imaging. Frank Friedersdorff reports no conflict of interest. Bernd Hamm reports having received consultancy honoraria from Canon Medical Imaging. Markus H. Lerchbaumer reports having received consultancy honoraria from Siemens Healthineers.

Abbreviations

ANOVA	analysis of variance
AUC	area under the curve
BMI	body mass index
CEUS	contrast-enhanced ultrasound
ceCT	contrast-enhanced computed tomography
ceMRI	contrast-enhanced magnetic resonance imaging
CI	confidence interval
IQR	interquartile range
ROC	receiver operating characteristics
SRM	small renal mass
US	ultrasound

References

1. Gill, I.S.; Aron, M.; Gervais, D.A.; Jewett, M.A.S. Clinical practice. Small renal mass. *N. Engl. J. Med.* **2010**, *362*, 624–634. [CrossRef]
2. Hara, A.K.; Johnson, C.D.; MacCarty, R.L.; Welch, T.J. Incidental extracolonic findings at CT colonography. *Radiology* **2000**, *215*, 353–357. [CrossRef]
3. Tada, S.; Yamagishi, J.; Kobayashi, H.; Hata, Y.; Kobari, T. The incidence of simple renal cyst by computed tomography. *Clin. Radiol.* **1983**, *34*, 437–439. [CrossRef]
4. Turner, R.M., 2nd; Morgan, T.M.; Jacobs, B.L. Epidemiology of the Small Renal Mass and the Treatment Disconnect Phenomenon. *Urol. Clin. N. Am.* **2017**, *44*, 147–154. [CrossRef] [PubMed]
5. Hollingsworth, J.M.; Miller, D.C.; Daignault, S.; Hollenbeck, B.K. Rising incidence of small renal masses: A need to reassess treatment effect. *J. Natl. Cancer Inst.* **2006**, *98*, 1331–1334. [CrossRef] [PubMed]
6. Patel, H.D.; Semerjian, A.; Gupta, M.; Pavlovich, C.P.; Johnson, M.H.; Gorin, M.A.; Allaf, M.E.; Pierorazio, P.M. Surgical removal of renal tumors with low metastatic potential based on clinical radiographic size: A systematic review of the literature. *Urol. Oncol.* **2019**, *37*, 519–524. [CrossRef] [PubMed]
7. Kutikov, A.; Fossett, L.K.; Ramchandani, P.; Tomaszewski, J.E.; Siegelman, E.S.; Banner, M.P.; Van Arsdalen, K.N.; Wein, A.J.; Malkowicz, S.B. Incidence of benign pathologic findings at partial nephrectomy for solitary renal mass presumed to be renal cell carcinoma on preoperative imaging. *Urology* **2006**, *68*, 737–740. [CrossRef] [PubMed]
8. Frank, I.; Blute, M.L.; Cheville, J.C.; Lohse, C.M.; Weaver, A.L.; Zincke, H. Solid renal tumors: An analysis of pathological features related to tumor size. *J. Urol.* **2003**, *170*, 2217–2220. [CrossRef]
9. Vogel, C.; Ziegelmuller, B.; Ljungberg, B.; Bensalah, K.; Bex, A.; Canfield, S.; Giles, R.H.; Hora, M.; Kuczyk, M.A.; Merseburger, A.S.; et al. Imaging in Suspected Renal-Cell Carcinoma: Systematic Review. *Clin. Genitourin. Cancer* **2019**, *17*, e345–e355. [CrossRef]
10. Rossi, S.H.; Prezzi, D.; Kelly-Morland, C.; Goh, V. Imaging for the diagnosis and response assessment of renal tumours. *World J. Urol.* **2018**, *36*, 1927–1942. [CrossRef]
11. Putz, F.J.; Verloh, N.; Erlmeier, A.; Schelker, R.C.; Schreyer, A.G.; Hautmann, M.G.; Stroszczynski, C.; Banas, B.; Jung, E.M. Influence of limited examination conditions on contrast-enhanced sonography for characterising liver lesions. *Clin. Hemorheol. Microcirc.* **2019**, *71*, 267–276. [CrossRef] [PubMed]
12. Sidhu, P.S.; Cantisani, V.; Dietrich, C.F.; Gilja, O.H.; Saftoiu, A.; Bartels, E.; Bertolotto, M.; Calliada, F.; Clevert, D.-A.D.-A.; Cosgrove, D.; et al. The EFSUMB Guidelines and Recommendations for the Clinical Practice of Contrast-Enhanced Ultrasound (CEUS) in Non-Hepatic Applications: Update 2017 (Long Version). *Ultraschall Med.* **2018**, *39*, e2–e44. [CrossRef] [PubMed]
13. Fetzer, D.T.; Rafailidis, V.; Peterson, C.; Grant, E.G.; Sidhu, P.; Barr, R.G. Artifacts in contrast-enhanced ultrasound: A pictorial essay. *Abdom. Radiol.* **2018**, *43*, 977–997. [CrossRef] [PubMed]
14. Dietrich, C.F.; Ignee, A.; Greis, C.; Cui, X.W.; Schreiber-Dietrich, D.G.; Hocke, M. Artifacts and pitfalls in contrast-enhanced ultrasound of the liver. *Ultraschall Med.* **2014**, *35*, 107–108. [CrossRef] [PubMed]
15. Piscaglia, F.; Bolondi, L. The safety of Sonovue in abdominal applications: Retrospective analysis of 23188 investigations. *Ultrasound Med. Biol.* **2006**, *32*, 1369–1375. [CrossRef]
16. Schwarze, V.; Marschner, C.; Negrão de Figueiredo, G.; Rübenthaler, J.; Clevert, D.-A. Single-Center Study: Evaluating the Diagnostic Performance and Safety of Contrast-Enhanced Ultrasound (CEUS) in Pregnant Women to Assess Hepatic Lesions. *Ultraschall Med.* **2020**, *41*, 29–35. [CrossRef]
17. Olson, M.C.; Abel, E.J.; Mankowski Gettle, L. Contrast-Enhanced Ultrasound in Renal Imaging and Intervention. *Curr. Urol. Rep.* **2019**, *20*, 73. [CrossRef]
18. Harvey, C.J.; Alsafi, A.; Kuzmich, S.; Ngo, A.; Papadopoulou, I.; Lakhani, A.; Berkowitz, Y.; Moser, S.; Sidhu, P.S.; Cosgrove, D.O. Role of US Contrast Agents in the Assessment of Indeterminate Solid and Cystic Lesions in Native and Transplant Kidneys. *Radiographics* **2015**, *35*, 1419–1430. [CrossRef]
19. Park, B.K.; Kim, B.; Kim, S.H.; Ko, K.; Lee, H.M.; Choi, H.Y. Assessment of cystic renal masses based on Bosniak classification: Comparison of CT and contrast-enhanced US. *Eur. J. Radiol.* **2007**, *61*, 310–314. [CrossRef]
20. Thorpe, S.; Salkovskis, P.M.; Dittner, A. Claustrophobia in MRI: The role of cognitions. *Magn. Reson. Imaging* **2008**, *26*, 1081–1088. [CrossRef]

21. Gulani, V.; Calamante, F.; Shellock, F.G.; Kanal, E.; Reeder, S.B. Gadolinium deposition in the brain: Summary of evidence and recommendations. *Lancet. Neurol.* **2017**, *16*, 564–570. [CrossRef]
22. Kahn, J.; Posch, H.; Steffen, I.G.; Geisel, D.; Bauknecht, C.; Liebig, T.; Denecke, T. Is There Long-term Signal Intensity Increase in the Central Nervous System on T1-weighted Images after MR Imaging with the Hepatospecific Contrast Agent Gadoxetic Acid? A Cross-sectional Study in 91 Patients. *Radiology* **2017**, *282*, 708–716. [CrossRef] [PubMed]
23. van der Molen, A.J.; Reimer, P.; Dekkers, I.A.; Bongartz, G.; Bellin, M.-F.; Bertolotto, M.; Clement, O.; Heinz-Peer, G.; Stacul, F.; Webb, J.A.W.; et al. Post-contrast acute kidney injury-Part 1: Definition, clinical features, incidence, role of contrast medium and risk factors: Recommendations for updated ESUR Contrast Medium Safety Committee guidelines. *Eur. Radiol.* **2018**, *28*, 2845–2855. [CrossRef] [PubMed]
24. Moos, S.I.; van Vemde, D.N.H.; Stoker, J.; Bipat, S. Contrast induced nephropathy in patients undergoing intravenous (IV) contrast enhanced computed tomography (CECT) and the relationship with risk factors: A meta-analysis. *Eur. J. Radiol.* **2013**, *82*, e387–e399. [CrossRef]
25. Kooiman, J.; Pasha, S.M.; Zondag, W.; Sijpkens, Y.W.J.; van der Molen, A.J.; Huisman, M.V.; Dekkers, O.M. Meta-analysis: Serum creatinine changes following contrast enhanced CT imaging. *Eur. J. Radiol.* **2012**, *81*, 2554–2561. [CrossRef]
26. Silverman, S.G.; Pedrosa, I.; Ellis, J.H.; Hindman, N.M.; Schieda, N.; Smith, A.D.; Remer, E.M.; Shinagare, A.B.; Curci, N.E.; Raman, S.S.; et al. Bosniak Classification of Cystic Renal Masses, Version 2019: An Update Proposal and Needs Assessment. *Radiology* **2019**, *292*, 475–488. [CrossRef]
27. Rogosnitzky, M.; Branch, S. Gadolinium-based contrast agent toxicity: A review of known and proposed mechanisms. *Biometals* **2016**, *29*, 365–376. [CrossRef]

Publisher's Note: MDPI stays neutral with regard to jurisdictional claims in published maps and institutional affiliations.

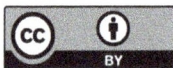

© 2020 by the authors. Licensee MDPI, Basel, Switzerland. This article is an open access article distributed under the terms and conditions of the Creative Commons Attribution (CC BY) license (http://creativecommons.org/licenses/by/4.0/).

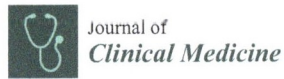

Article

Single-Site Sutureless Partial Nephrectomy for Small Exophytic Renal Tumors

Ching-Chia Li [1,2,3,4], Tsu-Ming Chien [1,2,3,*], Shu-Pin Huang [1,2], Hsin-Chih Yeh [4], Hsiang-Ying Lee [4], Hung-Lung Ke [1,2,3], Sheng-Chen Wen [1,2], Wei-Che Chang [1,2], Yung-Shun Juan [1,2,4], Yii-Her Chou [1,2,3] and Wen-Jeng Wu [1,2,3,*]

1. Department of Urology, Kaohsiung Medical University Hospital, Kaohsiung 80756, Taiwan; ccli1010@hotmail.com (C.-C.L.); shpihu73@gmail.com (S.-P.H.); hunglungke@yahoo.com.tw (H.-L.K.); CARL0815@gmail.com (S.-C.W.); u96000018@kmu.edu.tw (W.-C.C.); juanuro@gmail.com (Y.-S.J.); yihech@kmu.edu.tw (Y.-H.C.)
2. Department of Urology, Faculty of Medicine, College of Medicine, Kaohsiung Medical University, Kaohsiung 80756, Taiwan
3. Graduate Institute of Clinical Medicine, College of Medicine, Kaohsiung Medical University, Kaohsiung 80756, Taiwan
4. Department of Urology, Kaohsiung Municipal Ta-Tung Hospital, Kaohsiung 80145, Taiwan; patrick1201.tw@yahoo.com.tw (H.-C.Y.); ashum1009@hotmail.com (H.-Y.L.)
* Correspondence: slaochain@gmail.com (T.-M.C.); wejewu@kmu.edu.tw (W.-J.W.); Tel.: +886-7-320-8212 (T.-M.C. & W.-J.W.)

Received: 17 September 2020; Accepted: 10 November 2020; Published: 13 November 2020

Abstract: Partial nephrectomy (PN) is the standard procedure for most patients with localized renal cancer. Laparoscopy has become the preferred surgical approach to target this cancer, but the steep learning curve with laparoscopic PN (LPN) remains a concern. In LPN intracorporeal suturing, the operation time is further extended even under robot assistance, a step which prolongs warm ischemic time. Herein, we shared our experience to reduce the warm ischemia time, which allows surgeons to perform LPN more easily by using a combination of hemostatic agents to safely control parenchymal bleeding. Between 2015 and 2018, we enrolled 52 patients who underwent LPN in our hospital. Single-site sutureless LPN and traditional suture methods were performed in 33 and 19 patients, respectively. Preoperative, intra-operative, and postoperative variables were recorded. Renal function was evaluated by estimated glomerular filtration rate (eGFR) pre- and postoperatively. The average warm ischemia time (sutureless vs. suture group; 11.8 ± 3.9 vs. 21.2 ± 7.2 min, $p < 0.001$) and the operation time (167.9 ± 37.5 vs. 193.7 ± 42.5 min, $p = 0.035$) were significantly shorter in the sutureless group. In the sutureless group, only 2 patients suffered from massive urinary leakage (>200 mL/day) from the Jackson Pratt drainage tube, but the leakage spontaneously decreased within 7 days after surgery. eGFR and serum hemoglobin were not found to be significantly different pre- and postoperatively. All tumors were removed without a positive surgical margin. All patients were alive without recurrent tumors at mean postoperative follow-ups of 29.3 ± 12.2 months. Single-site sutureless LPN is a feasible surgical method for most patients with small exophytic renal cancer with excellent cosmetic results without affecting oncological results.

Keywords: partial nephrectomy; single site surgery; sutureless

1. Introduction

In 2009, the American Urological Association (AUA) [1] recommended partial nephrectomy (PN) as the reference standard treatment for most clinical T1 renal masses, even in individuals with a normal contralateral kidney, due to its similar efficacy to radical nephrectomy while also preserving kidney tissue. Since that time, a review of nephrectomy records submitted as part of the American Board of Urology surgeon certification/recertification process revealed that the use of PN has increased from 25% to 39% in all nephrectomies [2]. PN preserves kidney function better and limits long-term development of metabolic and cardiovascular disorders. The European Association of Urology has also considered PN the treatment of choice for T1b renal cell carcinoma (RCC) [3].

Open PN remains the gold standard procedure in most patients with localized renal cancer. Though no randomized controlled studies have compared the safety and oncological outcomes in terms of renal function and surgical margins, the steep learning curve with laparoscopic partial nephrectomy (LPN) remains a concern [4]. LPN is a technically demanding procedure, even under robotic assistance. Several important challenges, such as preventing perioperative bleeding, reaching hyperthermia after renal artery clamping, reducing warm ischemia time, and performing laparoscopic intracorporeal suturing, must be met during the operation. Despite the ability to achieve renal hyperthermia by delivering cold saline into the renal pelvis, the cooling effect is not qualified during laparoscopic surgery. Gill et al. [5] reported a novel method using ice slush around the kidney; however, this is difficult to replicate during the laparoscopic procedure. Because it is difficult to achieve renal hypothermia during LPN, it is important to reduce the warm ischemia time, which is understood to correlate with subsequent return of renal function [6]. Traditional clamping procedures require a significant warm ischemia time during the suturing process. Hemostatic suturing plays a vitally important role, even in the current era of early unclamping [7], selective clamping [8], and unclamping techniques [9–11]. With the introduction of hemostatic agents and improvements in surgical equipment allows for the resection of renal tumors without intracorporal suturing [12–16]. The suture method might also have contributed to the occurrence of pseudoaneurysms after the closure of renal defects [17]. Recently, there has been a growing application in laparoscopic single-site surgery that uses a single skin incision to gain access to the target operation site [15,16]. Single-site approach tries to minimize the rare port-related complications and fasten the postoperative recovery with excellent cosmetic results [15,16]. Robotic-assisted surgery is the new gold standard for uro-oncological surgery. However, the rigid instrumentation and the need for adaptation to the existing platform make the widespread use of these single- site surgeries difficult.

We previously shared our "pressure-cooker" method of performing LPN without intracorporeal suturing [12]. In the current study, we present our technique of single-site sutureless LPN. Our method is shown to reduce the warm ischemia time, and we believe that this technique allows surgeons to perform LPM more easily and effectively with fewer complications for those who lack experience in intracorporeal suturing.

2. Materials and Methods

2.1. Patient

In total, 116 consecutive patients with a renal tumor between 2015 and 2018 were sampled at the Kaohsiung Medical University Hospital in Kaohsiung, Taiwan. We firstly excluded metastatic tumors ($N = 29$). Patients with T2 renal tumor were also excluded ($N = 31$). Moreover, we excluded the two follow-up patients we lost, as well as the patient with a bilateral tumor. A total of 52 patients underwent LPN and were included in the current study. Single-site sutureless LPN and traditional suture methods were performed in 33 and 19 patients, respectively. All patients were informed of the potential complications and risks of the novel techniques. The study was conducted according to the principles of the Declaration of Helsinki and supervised by the local Ethics Committee of the Kaohsiung Medical University Hospital (KMUHIRB-E(I)-20180174). Written informed consent was obtained from all patients prior to their enrollment in the study. Patients with localized renal parenchymal tumor (stage T1N0M0) without endophytic properties or tumor located <4 mm from the collecting system were included. We excluded patients with suspected lymph node or distant metastasis. We quantified the anatomical characteristics of the renal masses using the RENAL nephrometry score [18]. In total, 52 patients who underwent LPN were enrolled in the study and had at least a one year follow-up (Figure 1). The authors confirmed that all ongoing and related trials for this intervention were registered.

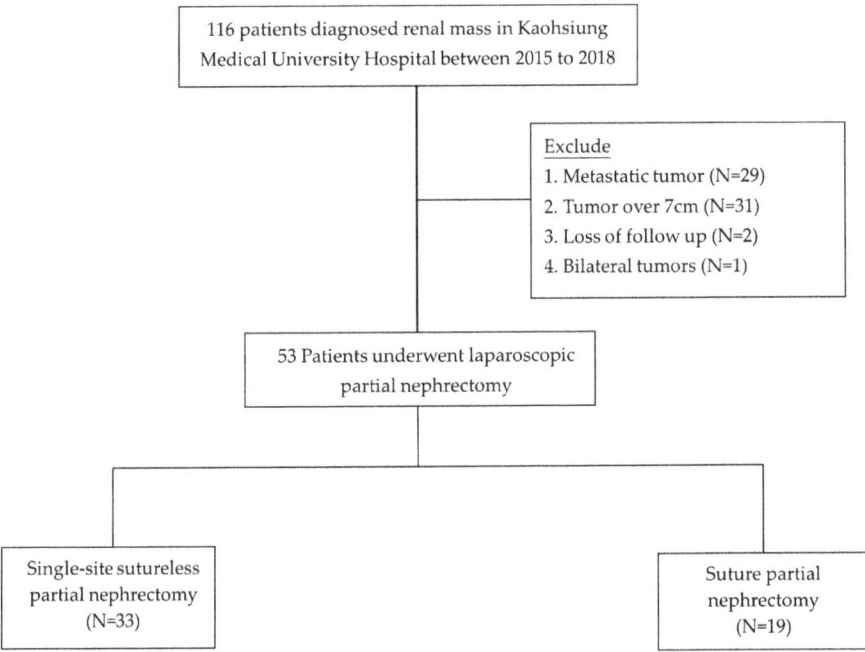

Figure 1. Patient enrollment for patients with renal tumor underwent surgical interventions.

2.2. Approach

We previously published an article that reported our basic sutureless LPN method [12]. Patients were placed in flank position with the lesion site elevated to 90 degrees. The surgeon and assistant stood facing the patient's back. The length of the skin incision was approximately 2.5–3.5 cm according to the tumor diameter. The port incision was made just below the 12th rib in the posterior axillary line. All procedures were performed using the retroperitoneal approach. A balloon dilator was used to create the retroperitoneal space, which was entered via the exposed thoracolumbar fascia, irrespective of their location. We used the LagiPort (Lagis, Inc., Taichung, Taiwan), a multi-instrument access port designed especially for single-site LPN (Figure 2). Gerota's fascia was dissected anteriorly and posteriorly. Next, an incision was made to mobilize the kidney from the perirenal fat, revealing the renal artery and primary tumor. If the tumor margin was not clear, intraoperative ultrasonography was used to better visualize the tumor margin. A fat pad from the perirenal space was prepared and was located as far away from the tumor as possible.

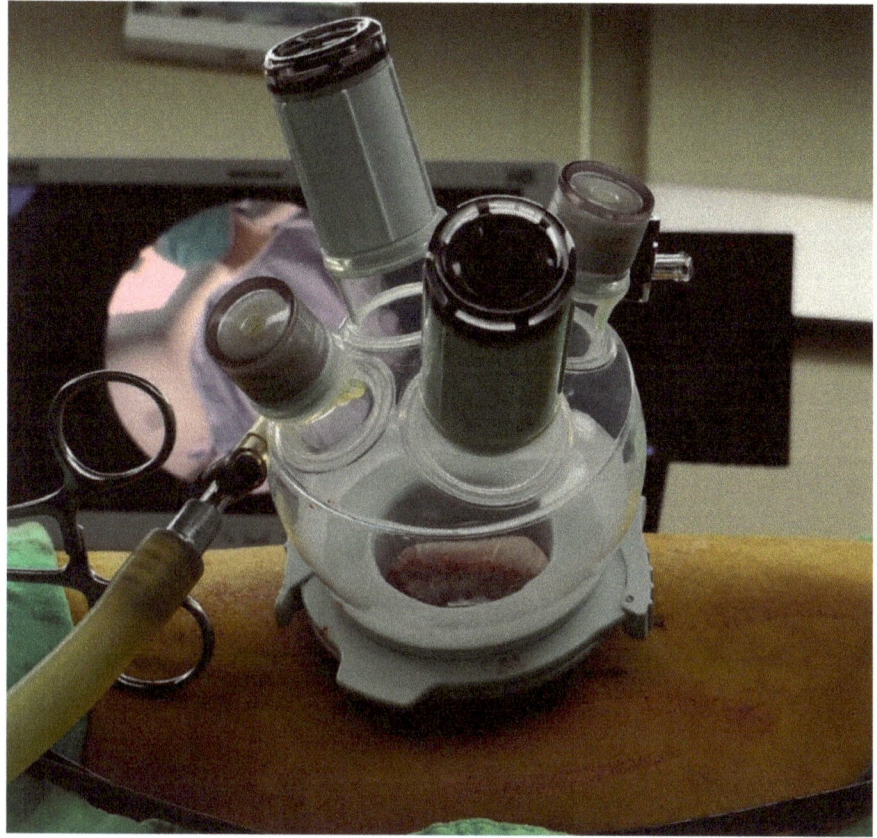

Figure 2. Placement of the LagiPort trocar.

2.3. Tumor Excision: The "Pressure Cooker" Method

In the selective renal artery non-clamping patients, a harmonic scalpel was used to remove the tumor, leaving a 0.5 to 1 cm safety margin. In the renal clamping group, the tumor was excised using laparoscopic scissors with bulldog clamps. Vascular disruption with excision was extensively fulgurated. For this procedure, we used monopolar coagulation via laparoscopic scissors to seal off the cross-section of renal calyx or pelvis if any collecting system disruptions are noted. After tumor removal, a hemostatic matrix (FloSeal; Baxter Healthcare, Zurich, Switzerland) was placed into the renal cavity, and a fibrin sealant (Tisseel; Baxter) was injected to cover the entire hemostatic matrix and the surrounding normal renal tissue. At the end of the surgery, the fat pad was placed to cover all areas coated with fibrin sealant, and the bulldog clamp was detached. The fat pad covering should be accomplished within 20 s to prevent solidifying of the fibrin sealant. The fat pad adhered to the periphery of the incision field, and the hemostatic matrix was "cooked" and closed off underneath. After the gelatin matrix and thrombin component were combined, the hemostatic matrix expanded around 20% of the volume upon contact with blood or urine. This reaction occurred soon after removing the bulldog clamp. The hemostatic matrix was engorged within the airtight space covered by the fat pad just like a "pressure cooker," causing extra external pressure to compress the postoperative bleeding (Figure 3). The tumor specimen was removed directly through the port using a laparoscopic grasper. We routinely placed a drainage tube after the surgery.

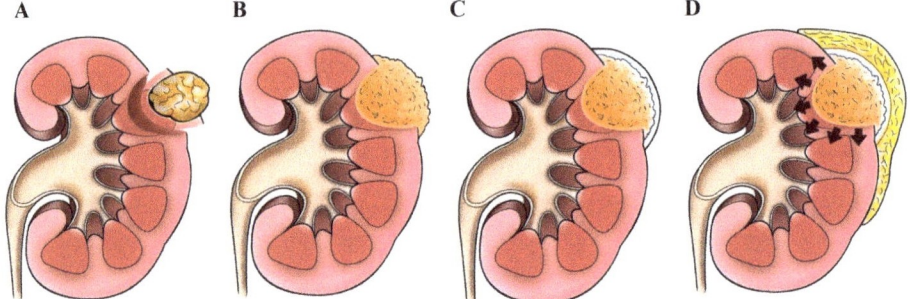

Figure 3. (**A**) A defect after tumor was removed. (**B**) FloSeal was placed into the defect of the kidney. (**C**) Tisseel was then injected to cover the whole hemostatic matrix and surrounding normal kidney surface. (**D**) A fat pad was placed on the top the field covered with Tisseel. FloSeal will swell in the airtight space, like a "pressure cooker".

2.4. Statistical Methods

All values are expressed as a mean ± standard deviation. Differences between categorical parameters were assessed using a χ^2 or Fisher's exact test, as appropriate. A Fisher's exact test was used when the sample number was small. Continuous parameters were assessed by using a *t*-test or Mann–Whitney–Wilcoxon test. The threshold for statistical significance was set at $p < 0.05$. SPSS 20.0J (SPSS Inc., Chicago, IL, USA) and used for all statistical analyses.

3. Results

3.1. Study Population

The preoperative data are shown in Table 1. The average patient age was older in the sutureless group. Twenty-four patients (46.1%) were female. The patient population was generally non-obese with a mean body mass index of 26.8 ± 3.3 (range: 21.9–38.1). Preoperative American Society of Anesthesiologists and Eastern Cooperative Oncology Group scores were 1.2 ± 0.4 (range: 1.0–2.0) and 0.3 ± 0.4 (range: 0–1), respectively. Twenty-nine patients had a left-sided renal mass. The average tumor size was 2.6 ± 1.1 cm (range: 1.5–5.0 cm). The mean R.E.N.A.L. nephrometry score [18] was 5.8 ± 1.5 (range: 4.0–9.0).

Table 1. Preoperative data on patients who underwent surgery.

Preoperative Variable	Total (N = 52)	Sutureless Group (N = 33)	Suture Group (N = 19)	*p* Value
Age (Mean ± SD), years	57.1 ± 10.7	59.7 ± 11.1	52.5 ± 8.5	0.013
Gender (female/male ratio)	0.46	0.48	0.42	0.715
BMI (Mean ± SD), kg/m^2	26.8 ± 3.3	26.8 ± 3.2	26.7 ± 3.6	0.917
Left/right kidney	29/23	18/15	11/9	0.974
ASA score (Mean ± SD)	1.2 ± 0.4	1.2 ± 0.4	1.3 ± 0.5	0.366
ECOG score (Mean ± SD)	0.3 ± 0.4	0.3 ± 0.5	0.3 ± 0.4	0.751
Tumor size (Mean ± SD), cm	2.6 ± 1.1	2.7 ± 1.1	2.5 ± 1.0	0.538
R.E.N.A.L. score (Mean ± SD)	5.8 ± 1.5	5.7 ± 1.5	5.9 ± 1.7	0.626
Preoperative eGFR, mL/min/m^2	79.7 ± 21.1	76.6 ± 22.4	85.1 ± 18.1	0.146
Preoperative hemoglobin, g/dL	13.9 ± 1.4	13.9 ± 1.3	14.0 ± 1.5	0.884

3.2. Surgical Outcomes

The average operation time was 177.3 ± 40.9 min (range: 100–250 min). To achieve renal hilar control, the clampless method was used in 7 patients due to tumors in exophytic locations or the majority of tumors had a distinct fibrotic capsule. Bulldog clamps were used for temporary renal artery occlusion in the remaining 27 patients. The average warm ischemia time was 15.5 ± 7.1 min (range: 8–26 min). The renal clamping strategy was made according to the surgeon, preoperative imaging, intraoperative findings, and intraoperative ultrasound. Mean estimated blood loss was 102.4 ± 97.2 mL (range: 10.0–430.0 mL). Only 3 patients required a perioperative blood transfusion due to large tumor burden. Conversion to conventional laparoscopy or open surgery was not necessary (Table 2). We did not perform the renal cooling technique. After the operation, the renal tumor was removed from the single-site wound. In total, 5 patients had obvious collecting system disruption during the procedures. We did not perform reconstruction of the collecting system. Only 2 patients suffered from massive urinary leakage (>200 mL/day) from the Jackson Pratt drainage tube (Table 3), but the leakage spontaneously decreased within 7 days after the surgery without requiring additional surgery. The mean length of hospital stay was 5.6 ± 1.3 days. The average warm ischemia time (sutureless vs. suture group; 11.8 ± 3.9 vs. 21.2 ± 7.2 min, $p < 0.001$) and the operation time (167.9 ± 37.5 vs. 193.7 ± 42.5 min, $p = 0.035$) were significantly shorter in the sutureless group.

Table 2. Intraoperative and postoperative data on patients who underwent surgery.

Intra-Operative and Postoperative Variable	Total (N = 52)	Sutureless Group (N = 33)	Suture Group (N = 19)	p Value
Operation time (Mean ± SD), min	177.3 ± 40.9	167.9 ± 37.5	193.7 ± 42.5	0.035
Renal artery control (clamped)	45 (86.5%)	27 (81.8%)	18 (94.7%)	0.189
Warm ischemia time (Mean ± SD), min	15.5 ± 7.1	11.8 ± 3.9	21.2 ± 7.2	<0.001
Blood loss (Mean ± SD), mL	102.4 ± 97.2	104.0 ± 105.8	99.7 ± 83.6	0.881
Transfusion	3 (5.8%)	1 (3.0%)	2 (10.5%)	0.264
Conversion to conventional laparoscopy	0	0	0	
Hospital stay (Mean ± SD), day	5.6 ± 1.3	5.6 ± 1.5	5.5 ± 1.6	0.848
Postoperative eGFR, mL/min/m^2	70.3 ± 25.2	69.6 ± 24.3	72.2 ± 21.8	0.340
Postoperative hemoglobin, g/dL	13.4 ± 1.4	13.3 ± 1.3	13.5 ± 1.5	0.642
Skin incision (Mean ± SD), cm	2.8 ± 1.2	2.8 ± 1.1	2.9 ± 1.4	0.771

Table 3. Histopathological and follow-up results on patients who underwent surgery.

Histopathological Variable	Total (N = 52)	Sutureless Group (N = 33)	Suture Group (N = 19)
Clear cell RCC			
pT1a	22 (42.3%)	14 (42.4%)	8 (42.1%)
pT1b	6 (11.5%)	4 (12.1%)	2 (10.5%)
Papillary RCC			
pT1a	5 (9.6%)	3 (9.1%)	2 (10.5%)
Chromophobe RCC			
pT1a	1 (1.9%)	1 (3.0%)	0 (0%)
Angiomyolipoma	10 (19.2%)	8 (24.2%)	2 (10.5%)
Oncocytoma	5 (9.6%)	3 (9.1%)	2 (10.5%)
Complications			
Prolong urine leakage	2 (3.8%)	2 (6.1%)	0 (0%)
Positive surgical margin	2 (3.8%)	2 (6.1%)	0 (0%)
Cancer recurrence	0 (0%)	0 (0%)	0 (0%)
Duration of follow-up (Mean ± SD), months	29.3 ± 12.2	27.5 ± 10.4	35.2 ± 14.3

RCC: Renal cell carcinoma.

3.3. Histopathological Outcome

The pathological results revealed clear cell RCC in 28 patients (53.8%; pT1a in 22 and pT1b in 6), angiomyolipoma in 10 (19.2%), oncocytoma in 5 (9.6%), papillary RCC in 5 (9.6%; all pT1a), and chromophobe RCC in 1 (1.9%; pT1a) (Table 3). One oncocytoma and one angiomyolipoma patient with positive surgical margins received a close follow-up ultrasound and computed tomography scans. Neither the residual tumor nor recurrence were observed in an imaging study after a 36 month follow-up. All patients were alive without recurrent tumors at a mean postoperative follow-up of 29.3 ± 12.2 months (range: 12.0–46.0 months).

3.4. Renal Function and Hemoglobin Level

The preoperative and postoperative estimated glomerular filtration rate (eGFR) was 79.7 ± 21.1 and 70.3 ± 25.2, respectively. There was no significant decrease in eGFR level ($p = 0.592$). A mild decrease in hemoglobin level was observed (preoperative vs postoperative; 13.9 ± 1.4 vs 13.4 ± 1.4; $p = 0.04$) (Tables 2 and 3). Notably, the average skin incision was 2.8 ± 1.2 cm with excellent cosmetic outcomes.

4. Discussion

PN was initially reported in 1993, wherein McDougall et al. [19] first reported a wedge resection technique for the removal of small, low-stage renal masses via LPN. Since then, LPN has been increasingly used due to refined laparoscopic suturing techniques and the availability of hemosealant substances. Although no randomized study has compared safety and oncological outcomes between LPN and the open technique, the main concern with LPN has always been the steep learning curve [4]. Stifelman el al. [20] reported the first robotic-assisted (RA) PN in 2005, demonstrating that this approach allowed for accurate lesion resection and easier reconstruction of the renal defect. A recent U.S. study [21] using the Nationwide Inpatient Sample database determined practice patterns and perioperative outcomes of open and minimally invasive PN, revealing that RAPN is currently performed more commonly than is LPN. Conversely, LPN is more widely used (69.8%) in minimally invasive procedures compared to RAPN (30.2%) in the U.K [22]. A recent meta-analysis [23] combining 4919 patients from 25 studies (RAPN in 2681 and LPN in 2238) revealed no significant differences between the 2 groups in terms of age, sex, laterality, and final malignant pathology; however, the tumor was larger, with higher mean R.E.N.A.L. nephrometry scores in the former group. Patients treated with RAPN had a decreased likelihood of conversion to open surgery compared to those treated with LPN. RAPN also was associated with reduced complications, fewer positive margins, and shorter warm ischemia time [23]. Potential disadvantages of RAPN included cost, training, setup time, and lack of tactile sensation or haptics. The robotic procedure had lower odds of advantages compared to LPN, except for hospital charges. Nonetheless, LPN still has a competitive value in patients with small exophytic renal tumors. The major concern with LPN is the learning curve. Our technique provides a feasible method without the use of intracorporeal suturing and achieves excellent functional outcomes without affecting oncological results. At our institution, we started performing LPN in 2003 and single-site LPN in 2013. We have also performed RAPN for large renal tumors since 2015. In recent years, single-site LPN has been our standard operation for patients with small renal masses. For those with larger tumors, open and RAPN are two of our most utilized surgical procedures.

Our study identified 5 patients with obvious disruption of the collecting system. We did not perform traditional suture repair of the collecting system. Ploussard et al. [24] showed that even after deep one-third PN, the combinations of FloSeal and Tisseel appeared to sufficiently control the major medullary vascular injuries and replace the conventional deep medullary sutures without compromising operative outcomes in a pig model. We previously described our methods using combinations of hemostatic agents with a fat pad around the outer layer of the kidney. The fat pad encapsulated the hemostatic agents within the tumor-excised cavity, supplementing structural support of the expanding and swelling action of FloSeal after it interacts with blood or urine from within. The extra external pressure provided by the fat pad acts in theory like a "pressure cooker" in preventing postoperative bleeding. The suture procedure may occlude unnecessary vessels at the suture site, leading to areas of kidney necrosis in the region. By decreasing the risk of unnecessary segmental vessel occlusion, the potential advantages may be noted during functional and vascular follow-up examinations.

Pathologic difference is an important prognostic factor for renal tumor [25]. Exophytic renal tumors tended to be associated with lower pathologic grade and the presence of papillary renal cell carcinoma subtype when compared with endophytic renal tumors [25]. Papillary renal carcinoma is reported to have better outcomes than clear cell renal cell carcinoma in patients without metastases [26]. Furthermore, the presence of an angular interface with the normal renal parenchyma is strongly related to benignity in an exophytic renal mass. Thus, a simple assessment of the angular interface sign can be considered as an additional parameter to characterize exophytic renal masses [27]. Optimal follow-up or therapy for patients with renal tumors should be assigned according to the tumor stage and subtype. The aforementioned information may be useful when small tumors are being considered for watchful waiting or ablative therapies.

The most important factor in preserving renal function during PN is the percent of nephron mass preserved [6,28–30]. In our series, one of our main findings relates to nephron mass preservation, which is of primary importance for functional recovery, consistent with reports from other studies that eGFR of small renal cancer was not significantly different pre- and postoperatively [10,11]. Traditionally, LPN relies on clamping the main artery, with ischemia time considered to correlate with postoperative renal function. Gill et al. [5] shared a novel technique of laparoscopic renal hypothermia with intracorporeal ice slush during LPN. However, this cooling procedure was not easy to replicate during laparoscopic surgery; therefore, it is important to reduce the warm ischemia time. A threshold may exist after the damage from ischemia begins. Thompson et al. [6] demonstrated that every minute is important, and 25 min was considered a safe threshold in patients with a solitary kidney. Lane et al. [30] evaluated early and late renal functional outcomes in 1132 patients with 2 functioning kidneys, showing that a warm ischemia time of <20 min is not associated with clinically relevant functional loss compared to that of alternative techniques. Gill et al. [9] was the first to describe a technique of "zero ischemia," which focused special attention on selective branch microdissection of renal vessels in the renal sinus; transient, pharmacologically induced blood pressure reduction timed to coincide precisely with excision of the deep part of the tumor; laparoscopic ultrasound to score the proposed resection margin; and clip ligation of any specific tertiary or quaternary renal artery branches supplying the tumor. The effort to minimize ischemia is accompanied by increased blood loss during the procedure. The potential impact on the surgical margin may be influenced by the lack of a clear operative field, which may bring surgical challenges for inexperienced operators, especially in larger renal tumors [31]. A current review paper [31] argued that newer strategies focusing on selective clamping and non-clamping can make a complex surgery even more challenging, which may serve to limit the widespread use of LPN for management of renal cancers. We believe that our technique should be used in single-site sutureless LPN to improve not only the warm ischemia time but also allows surgeons to perform LPM more easily and more effectively.

Our study has several limitations. First, this was not a randomized prospective analysis and was composed of a relatively small cohort. An important selection bias might have resulted in satisfied surgical outcomes due to all participants were patients with exophytic renal tumors. The use of this technique for endophytic tumor still needs to be explored. Our method allows surgeons to perform LPN more easily and effectively with fewer complications compared to the open method.

5. Conclusions

In conclusion, single-site sutureless LPN is a feasible surgical method for most patients with small exophytic renal cancer with excellent cosmetic results without affecting oncological results. Further prospective studies with longer follow-up are needed to observe the oncological safety of the technique.

Author Contributions: Conceptualization, C.-C.L. and W.-J.W.; methodology, T.-M.C. and W.-C.C.; data curation, S.-P.H., H.-C.Y., H.-Y.L., H.-L.K., S.-C.W. and Y.-S.J.; writing—original draft preparation, T.-M.C. and C.-C.L.; writing—review and editing, Y.-H.C. and W.-J.W.; supervision, W.-J.W. All authors have read and agreed to the published version of the manuscript.

Funding: This research received no external funding.

Acknowledgments: The authors gratefully acknowledge the assistance of all the members in our group.

Conflicts of Interest: The authors declare that they have no conflict of interest.

References

1. Campbell, S.C.; Novick, A.C.; Belldegrun, A.; Blute, M.L.; Chow, G.K.; Derweesh, I.H.; Faraday, M.M.; Kaouk, J.H.; Leveillee, R.J.; Matin, S.F.; et al. Guideline for management of the clinical T1 renal mass. *J. Urol.* **2009**, *182*, 1271–1279. [CrossRef] [PubMed]
2. Sorokin, I.; Feustel, P.J.; O'Malley, R.L. National utilization of partial nephrectomy pre- and post- AUA Guidelines: Is this as good as it gets? *Clin. Genitourin. Cancer* **2017**, *15*, 591–597. [CrossRef] [PubMed]
3. Ljungberg, B.; Hanbury, D.C.; Kuczyk, M.A.; Merseburger, A.S.; Mulders, P.F.; Patard, J.J.; Sinescu, I.C. Renal cell carcinoma guideline. *Eur. Urol.* **2007**, *51*, 1502–1510. [CrossRef] [PubMed]
4. Springer, C.; Hoda, M.R.; Fajkovic, H.; Pini, G.; Mohammed, N.; Fornara, P.; Greco, F. Laparoscopic vs open partial nephrectomy for T1 renal tumours: Evaluation of long-term oncological and functional outcomes in 340 patients. *BJU Int.* **2013**, *111*, 281–288. [CrossRef]
5. Gill, I.S.; Abreu, S.C.; Desai, M.M.; Steinberg, A.P.; Ramani, A.P.; Ng, C.; Banks, K.; Novick ACKaouk, J.H. Laparoscopic ice slush renal hypothermia for partial nephrectomy: The initial experience. *J. Urol.* **2003**, *170*, 52–56. [CrossRef]
6. Thompson, R.H.; Lane, B.R.; Lohse, C.M.; Leibovich, B.C.; Fergany, A.; Frank, I.; Gill, I.S.; Blute, M.L.; Campbell, S.C. Every minute counts when the renal hilum is clamped during partial nephrectomy. *Eur. Urol.* **2010**, *58*, 340–345. [CrossRef]
7. Baumert, H.; Ballaro, A.; Shah, N.; Mansouri, D.; Zafar, N.; Molinié, V.; Neal, D. Reducing warm ischaemia time during laparoscopic partial nephrectomy: A prospective comparison of two renal closure techniques. *Eur. Urol.* **2007**, *52*, 1164–1169. [CrossRef]
8. Peyronnet, B.; Baumert, H.; Mathieu, R.; Masson-Lecomte, A.; Grassano, Y.; Roumiguié, M.; Massoud, W.; Abd El Fattah, V.; Bruyère, F.; Droupy, S.; et al. Early unclamping technique during robot-assisted laparoscopic partial nephrectomy can minimise warm ischaemia without increasing morbidity. *BJU Int.* **2014**, *114*, 741–747. [CrossRef]
9. Gill, I.S.; Eisenberg, M.S.; Aron, M.; Berger, A.; Ukimura, O.; Patil, M.B.; Campese, V.; Thangathurai, D.; Desai, M.M. "Zero ischemia" partial nephrectomy: Novel laparoscopic and robotic technique. *Eur. Urol.* **2011**, *59*, 128–134. [CrossRef]
10. Dell'Atti, L.; Scarcella, S.; Manno, S.; Polito, M.; Galosi, A.B. Approach for renal tumors with low nephrometry score through unclamped sutureless laparoscopic enucleation technique: Functional and oncologic outcomes. *Clin. Genitourin. Cancer* **2018**, *16*, e1251–e1256. [CrossRef]
11. Springer, C.; Veneziano, D.; Wimpissinger, F.; Inferrera, A.; Fornara, P.; Greco, F. Clampless laparoendoscopic single-site partial nephrectomy for renal cancer with low PADUA score: Technique and surgical outcomes. *BJU Int.* **2013**, *111*, 1091–1098. [CrossRef] [PubMed]
12. Li, C.C.; Yeh, H.C.; Lee, H.Y.; Li, W.M.; Ke, H.L.; Hsu, A.H.S.; Lee, M.H.; Tsai, C.C.; Chueh, K.S.; Huang, C.N.; et al. Laparoscopic partial nephrectomy without intracorporeal suturing. *Surg. Endosc.* **2016**, *30*, 1585–1591. [CrossRef] [PubMed]
13. Simone, G.; Papalia, R.; Guaglianone, S.; Gallucci, M. 'Zero ischaemia', sutureless laparoscopic partial nephrectomy for renal tumours with a low nephrometry score. *BJU Int.* **2012**, *110*, 124–130. [CrossRef] [PubMed]
14. Ota, T.; Komori, H.; Rii, J.; Ochi, A.; Suzuki, K.; Shiga, N.; Nishiyama, H. Soft coagulation in partial nephrectomy without renorrhaphy: Feasibility of a new technique and early outcomes. *Int. J. Urol.* **2014**, *21*, 244–247. [CrossRef] [PubMed]
15. Cindolo, L.; Berardinelli, F.; Gidaro, S.; Schips, L. Laparoendoscopic single-site partial nephrectomy without ischemia. *J. Endourol.* **2010**, *24*, 1997–2002. [CrossRef] [PubMed]
16. Kihara, K.; Koga, F.; Fujii, Y.; Masuda, H.; Tatokoro, M.; Yokoyama, M.; Matsuoka, Y.; Numao, N.; Ishioka, J.; Saito, K. Gasless laparoendoscopic single-port clampless sutureless partial nephrectomy for peripheral renal tumors: Perioperative outcomes. *Int. J. Urol.* **2015**, *22*, 349–355. [CrossRef]
17. Jain, S.; Nyirenda, T.; Yates, J.; Munver, R.J. Incidence of renal artery pseudoaneurysm following open and minimally invasive partial nephrectomy: A systematic review and comparative analysis. *J. Urol.* **2013**, *189*, 1643–1648. [CrossRef]
18. Kutikov, A.; Uzzo, R.G. The, R.E.N.A.L. nephrometry score: A comprehensive standardized system for quantitating renal tumor size, location and depth. *J. Urol.* **2009**, *182*, 844–853. [CrossRef]

19. McDougall, E.M.; Clayman, R.V.; Anderson, K. Laparoscopic wedge resection of a renal tumor: Initial experience. *J. Laparoendosc. Surg.* **1993**, *3*, 577–581. [CrossRef]
20. Stifelman, M.D.; Caruso, R.P.; Nieder, A.M.; Taneja, S.S. Robot-assisted Laparoscopic Partial Nephrectomy. *J. Soc. Laparoendosc. Surg.* **2005**, *9*, 83–86.
21. Ghani, K.R.; Sukumar, S.; Sammon, J.D.; Rogers, C.G.; Trinh, Q.D.; Menon, M. Practice patterns and outcomes of open and minimally invasive partial nephrectomy since the introduction of robotic partial nephrectomy: Results from the nationwide inpatient sample. *J. Urol.* **2014**, *191*, 907–912. [CrossRef] [PubMed]
22. Hadjipavlou, M.; Khan, F.; Fowler, S.; Joyce, A.; Keeley, F.X.; Sriprasad, S. BAUS Sections of Endourology and Oncology. Partial vs radical nephrectomy for T1 renal tumours: An analysis from the British Association of Urological Surgeons Nephrectomy Audit. *BJU Int.* **2016**, *117*, 62–71. [CrossRef] [PubMed]
23. Leow, J.J.; Heah, N.H.; Chang, S.L.; Chong, Y.L.; Png, K.S. Outcomes of robotic versus laparoscopic partial nephrectomy: An updated meta-analysis of 4,919 patients. *J. Urol.* **2016**, *196*, 1371–1377. [CrossRef] [PubMed]
24. Ploussard, G.; Haddad, R.; Loutochin, O.; Bera, R.; Cabrera, T.; Malibari, N.; Scarlata, E.; Derbekyan, V.; Bladou, F.; Anidjar, M. A combination of hemostatic agents may safely replace deep medullary suture during laparoscopic partial nephrectomy in a pig model. *J. Urol.* **2015**, *193*, 318–324. [CrossRef] [PubMed]
25. Lipke, M.C.; Ha, S.P.; Fischer, C.D.; Rydberg, J.; Bonsib, S.M.; Sundaram, C.P. Pathologic characteristics of exophytic renal masses. *J. Endourol.* **2007**, *21*, 1489–1491. [CrossRef] [PubMed]
26. Deng, J.; Li, L.; Xia, H.; Guo, J.; Wu, X.; Yang, X.; Hong, Y.; Chen, Q.; Hu, J. A comparison of the prognosis of papillary and clear cell renal cell carcinoma: Evidence from a meta-analysis. *Medicine (Baltimore)* **2019**, *98*, e16309. [CrossRef] [PubMed]
27. Verma, S.K.; Mitchell, D.G.; Yang, R.; Roth, C.G.; O'Kane, P.; Verma, M.; Parker, L. Exophytic renal masses: Angular interface with renal parenchyma for distinguishing benign from malignant lesions at MR imaging. *Radiology* **2010**, *255*, 501–507. [CrossRef]
28. Zhang, Z.; Zhao, J.; Dong, W.; Remer, E.; Li, J.; Demirjian, S.; Zabell, J.; Campbell, S.C. Acute kidney injury after partial nephrectomy: Role of parenchymal mass reduction and ischemia and impact on subsequent functional recovery. *Eur. Urol.* **2016**, *69*, 745–752. [CrossRef]
29. Rosen, D.C.; Kannappan, M.; Paulucci, D.J.; Beksac, A.T.; Attalla, K.; Abaza, R.; Eun, D.D.; Bhandari, A.; Hemal, A.K.; Porter, J.; et al. Reevaluating warm ischemia time as a predictor of renal function outcomes after robotic partial nephrectomy. *Urology* **2018**, *120*, 156–161. [CrossRef]
30. Lane, B.R.; Gill, I.S.; Fergany, A.F.; Larson, B.T.; Campbell, S.C. Limited warm ischemia during elective partial nephrectomy has only a marginal impact on renal functional outcomes. *J. Urol.* **2011**, *185*, 1598–1603. [CrossRef]
31. Mir, M.C.; Pavan, N.; Parekh, D.J. Current paradigm for ischemia in kidney surgery. *J. Urol.* **2016**, *195*, 1655–1663. [CrossRef] [PubMed]

Publisher's Note: MDPI stays neutral with regard to jurisdictional claims in published maps and institutional affiliations.

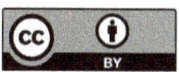

© 2020 by the authors. Licensee MDPI, Basel, Switzerland. This article is an open access article distributed under the terms and conditions of the Creative Commons Attribution (CC BY) license (http://creativecommons.org/licenses/by/4.0/).

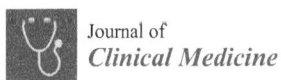

Review

Outcomes Related to Percutaneous Nephrostomies (PCN) in Malignancy-Associated Ureteric Obstruction: A Systematic Review of the Literature

Francesca J. New [1], Sally J. Deverill [2] and Bhaskar K. Somani [1,*]

[1] Department of Urology, University Hospital Southampton, Southampton SO16 6YD, UK; frankiejnew@gmail.com
[2] Department of Urology, Queen Alexandra Hospital, Portsmouth PO6 3LY, UK; s.deverill@doctors.org.uk
* Correspondence: bhaskar.somani@uhs.nhs.uk; Tel.: +44-238-1206-873

Abstract: Background: Malignant ureteric obstruction occurs in a variety of cancers and has been typically associated with a poor prognosis. Percutaneous nephrostomy (PCN) can potentially help increase patient longevity by establishing urinary drainage and treating renal failure. Our aim was to look at the outcomes of PCN in patients with advanced cancer and the impact on the patients' lifespan and quality of life. Materials and Methods: A literature review was carried out for articles from 2000 to 2020 on PCN in patients with advanced malignancies, using MEDLINE, EMBASE, Scopus, CINAHL, Cochrane Library, clinicaltrials.gov, and Google Scholar. All English-language articles reporting on a minimum of 20 patients who underwent PCN for malignancy-associated ureteric obstruction were included. Results: A total of 21 articles (1674 patients) met the inclusion criteria with a mean of 60.2 years (range: 21–102 years). PCN was performed for ureteric obstruction secondary to urological malignancies ($n = -633$, 37.8%), gynaecological malignancies ($n = 437$, 26.1%), colorectal and GI malignancies ($n = 216$, 12.9%), and other specified malignancies ($n = 205$, 12.2%). The reported mean survival times varied from 2 to 8.5 months post PCN insertion, with an average survival time of 5.6 months, which depended on the cancer type, stage, and previous treatment. Conclusions: Patients with advanced malignancies who need PCN tend to have a survival rate under 12 months and spend a large proportion of this time in the hospital. Although the advent of newer chemotherapy and immunotherapy options has changed the landscape of managing advanced cancer, decisions on nephrostomy must be balanced with their survival and quality of life, which must be discussed with the patient.

Keywords: prostate cancer; nephrostomy; quality of life; survival; decision making

1. Introduction

Malignancy-associated ureteric obstruction occurs in a variety of pelvic cancers, often as a late manifestation, which can be secondary to locally advanced disease or nodal metastases. Treatment consists of various options ranging from ureteric stent insertion (retrograde or antegrade), to percutaneous nephrostomy (PCN), to other forms of urinary diversion. While these procedures can help to improve renal function, they also risk complications and can have a profound effect on the quality of life (QoL). Stenting can consign the patient to stent symptoms (which may include frequency, urgency, pain, haematuria, and dysuria), and regular stent changes (typically every 6–12 months) under a general anaesthetic but is generally believed to be better for QoL than long-term PCN, although give the underlying disease this might be challenging [1].

Unfortunately, in the context of locally advanced pelvic cancers, there are often scenarios whereby a patient will start with a retrograde ureteric stent (RUS), but subsequently, as this fails, it necessitates PCN insertion. In the event that a RUS change or drainage fails, the decision to proceed with PCN often marks disease progression. Without treatment of malignant ureteric obstruction, the patient will deteriorate over time with symptoms of uraemia, fluid overload, electrolyte disturbances, flank pain, urinary infections, reduction in alertness, renal failure, and subsequent death [2]. Patients with advanced malignancies, who present with acute renal failure (ARF) due to malignant ureteric obstruction, are often poor surgical and/or anaesthetic candidates, and therefore PCN, which can be done under local anaesthesia (LA), is often preferred. Similarly, it is not always possible to insert primary retrograde stents in the context of locally advanced pelvic malignancies [3–5].

Percutaneous nephrostomy has a high rate of technical success; however, periprocedural complications can occur. These may include sepsis, bleeding or vascular injury, perirenal haematoma, and injury to surrounding structures such as colon, liver, and lung [3]. Furthermore, PCN can block, dislodge, develop line or component fracture, become infected, or colonised with bacteria, and patients can develop skin reactions, cellulitis, or abscesses [3]. Such complications can result in multiple readmissions to hospital, often needing a change in PCN, which can also significantly impact their QoL [1]. Emergency readmissions also happen if the PCN falls out completely, needing a new nephrostomy placement as a matter of urgency [6]. Patients with advanced cancers who develop infections secondary to nephrostomy are at a high risk of deterioration, especially if they are receiving immunosuppression such as chemotherapy or immunotherapy.

Most studies looking at malignancy-associated ureteric obstruction cover an extremely heterogenous population, with multiple different aetiologies and presentations. Treating malignant ureteric obstruction is an ever-changing landscape, and as newer cancer treatments become available, this continues to evolve. We aimed to review the quality of evidence available to date in this group of patients, establishing outcomes of PCN in malignancy-associated ureteric obstruction, assessing the risk of complications, life expectancy, QoL and potential indicators of favourable versus poorer outcomes.

2. Materials and Methods

2.1. Study Population

Population: Adults with malignancy-associated ureteric obstruction.
Intervention: Percutaneous nephrostomy.
Comparator: Not applicable for this study.
Outcome: Life expectancy, QoL, and outcomes related to PCN.

2.2. Inclusion Criteria

Studies reporting on patients with advanced malignancies with ureteric obstruction.
English-language studies reporting on a minimum of 20 patients.

2.3. Exclusion Criteria

PCN insertion for benign disease.
Studies that included primary ureteric stenting as the only treatment option.
Case reports, laboratory studies, or review articles.

2.4. Search Strategy and Study Selection

The systematic review was performed as per the Cochrane guidelines and the Preferred Reporting Items for Systematic Reviews and Meta-analyses (PRISMA) checklist [7]. The database searched were MEDLINE, EMBASE, Scopus, CINAHL, Cochrane Library, clinicaltrials.gov and Google Scholar from January 2000 to December 2020. The search terms included 'Nephrostomy', 'percutaneous nephrostomy', 'PCN', 'urinary drainage', 'stent', 'ureteric stent', 'prostate', 'ovarian', 'cervical', 'bowel', 'malignancies, malignancy or cancer', and 'pelvic, gynaecological, colorectal, urological'. Boolean operators (AND, OR) were used with the above search terms to refine the search. Two reviewers (S.D. and F.N.) independently identified all the studies that matched the inclusion criteria and any discrepancies were resolved by consensus with the senior author (BKS).

2.5. Data Extraction and Analysis

The primary outcome measures were complications after PCN, time spent in the hospital after PCN, and survival times after their first PCN. Secondary outcomes were QoL after PCN and differences in outcomes based on the cancer sub-type. Information was collected on the year of publication, type of malignancy, patient demographics, and outcomes of PCN. Data were collected using Microsoft Excel 2019 (version 19.0). A narrative review was done due to heterogeneity of the studies and data available.

3. Results

3.1. Literature Search and Included Studies

After an initial search of 110 articles, 21 studies (1674 patients) met the inclusion criteria for the final review (Figure 1) [3,6,8–26]. A full breakdown of the patient demographics can be seen in Table 1.

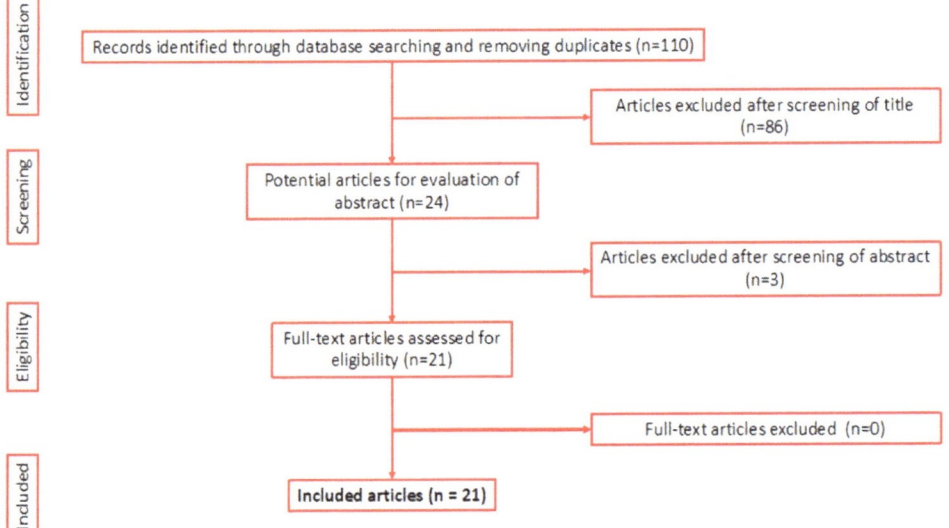

Figure 1. PRISMA flowchart of the included articles.

Table 1. Demographics, survival, cancer sub-type and time spent in the hospital.

Author/Year Published	Review Period	Mean Age (Range), Years	Total Number of Patients	Time Spent in Hospital after PCN	Survival Time after Insertion of PCN (Mean)	Malignancy Type	Number of Patients (Subgroup)	Breakdown of Survival per Cancer Type Post PCN Insertion (Months)
Ekici et al. [17], 2001	1987–2000	55 (25–76)	23	ND	4.9 months	Bladder	23	4.9
Little et al. [26], 2003	ND	69 (50–87)	31	46% of remaining life in hospital	7.7 months	Bladder Prostate Colorectal Gynaecological	16 8 4 3	ND
Tanaka et al. [16], 2004	1991–2003	69.2	33	70% remained in hospital post PCN	3 months	Urological Gynaecological Colorectal Upper GI Lung	8 8 8 8 1	3.0 3.0 5.5 1.5 2.5
Romero et al. [18], 2005	2000–2004	52	43	17% of their remaining life (58% readmission rate)	40% survival at 6 months, 24.2% survival at 1 year	Urological Gynaecological	15 28	40% survival at 6 months/10% at 1 year 44.6% survival at 6 months/38.45% at 1 year
Wilson et al. [19], 2005	1998–2001	68.1 (42–84)	32	29 days (81% readmission rate)	2.9 months	Urological Gynaecological Colorectal Breast	17 7 7 1	2.4 6.9 4.3 27.1
Harris et al. [20], 2006	2001–2004	75.9 (65–89)	26	51 days (Mean)	4.6 months	Prostate	26	2.9 months
Carrafiello et al. [13], 2006	2003–2006	65.7 (32–102)	201	ND	ND	ND	201	ND
Radecka et al. [3], 2006	1998–2002	73.1 (51–97)	151	ND	8.5 months	Prostate Bladder Gynaecological Colorectal other	55 43 11 16 26	6.9 17.6 31.2 4.3 10.1

Table 1. Cont.

Study	Years	Age (range)	N	Hospital stay	Survival	Cancer type	N	Survival detail
Aravantinos et al. [21], 2007	1996–2003	63 (40–86)	270	ND	67% of patients died in first 6 months post PCN	Bladder Prostate Gynae Colorectal other	54 54 54 54 54	8–270 days 22–723 days 7–269 days 9–272 days 8–280 days
Dienstmann et al. [22], 2008	2002–2006	44 (26–67)	50	22% of patients remained in hospital post PCN	2 months (median)	Cervical	50	2 months
Ishioka et al. [15], 2008	1995–2007	57 (31–85)	140	ND	3.2 months	Urological Gynaecological Colorectal other	13 36 34 57	ND
Nariculam et al. [23], 2009	1998–2006	71 (51–85)	25	ND	7.5 months	Prostate	25	7.5 months
Lienert et al. [10], 2009	2005–2007	71 (36–91) median	49	ND	5.8 months (median)	Urological Gynaecological Colorectal other	33 5 6 5	ND
Jalbani et al. [8], 2010	2004–2006	ND, (range 21–70)	40	ND	6.3 months (median)	Urological Gynaecological Colorectal other	15 17 3 5	14.3 11.3 1.2 ND
Plesinac-Karapandzic et al. [11], 2010	1996–2006	51 (28–85) median	117	ND	7 months (median)	Gynaecological	117	7 months
Malik et al. [14], 2010	2001–2009	68.67 (53–85)	28	ND	15 months	Prostate cancer	28	15 months
Misra et al. [12], 2013	2008	75.1 (54–87)	22	29% of life in hospital (100% readmission rate)	2.6 months	Urological Gynaecological Colorectal	18 2 2	33% survival at 6 months 100% survival at 6 months 0% survival at 6 months

Table 1. Cont.

Study	Years	Age	N	Follow-up	Cancer type	N	%
Alawneh et al. [9], 2016	2009–2013	Not reported	211	ND	Urological GI Other	122 61 28	5.5 5.2 3.6
De Souza et al. [24], 2016	2010–2012	48.2	45	ND	Cervical cancer	45	ND
McDevitt et al. [6], 2017	2011–2013	48 (21–79)	57	ND	Cervical Colorectal Prostate Bladder Lymphoma Ovarian other	26 6 6 4 3 3 9	ND
Folkard et al. [25], 2020	2015–2018	68.8 (30–93)	105	Median post procedure 14 days (1–104 days)	4.6 months	Bladder Prostate Colorectal Gynaecological Other	32 18 16 25 8	ND

3.2. Patient Characteristics

There were 1674 patients with a mean age of 60.2 years (range: 21–102 years), although two studies did not state the mean or median age [6,7], and two studies stated the median age [8,9]. The majority of studies were retrospective in nature (*n* = 17), with one prospective study [8] and four where the type of study was not specified (Table 1) [10–13].

PCN was performed for ureteric obstruction secondary to urological malignancies (*n* = 633, 37.8%), gynaecological malignancies (*n* = 437, 26.1%), colorectal and gastrointestinal (GI) malignancies (*n* = 216, 12.9%), and other specified malignancies (*n* = 205, 12.2%) (Table 1) [13]. Fourteen studies documented the length of survival post nephrostomy insertion for the different cancer subtypes [3,8,9,11,12,15–23].

3.3. Primary Outcomes

3.3.1. Survival Times after PCN

The reported mean survival time varied from 2.6 to 8.5 months post initial PCN insertion, with an average survival time of 5.9 months (Figure 2, Table 1). Five studies documented median survival time as 5.2 months (range: 2–7 months) [8–11,22], and three did not document the survival time post PCN insertion [6,13,24].

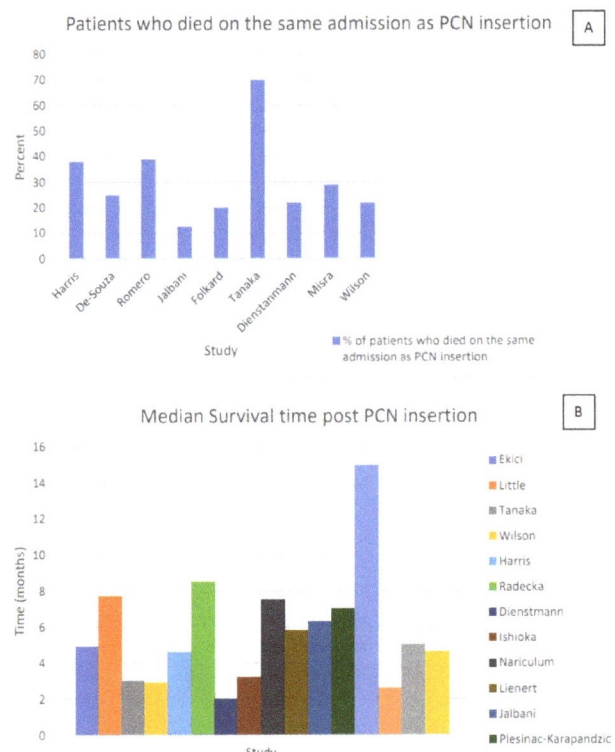

Figure 2. (**A**): Patients who died on the same admission as nephrostomy (PCN) insertion (**B**): Median survival post PCN insertion.

Romeo et al. [18] documented the survival times post PCN insertion with 40% dead at 6 months and a further 24.4% at 1 year, while Aravantious documented that 67% of the patients were dead within 6 months of a PCN insertion [21] (Table 1). A prostate cancer study by Nariculam and colleagues in 2009 found that the overall mean time to death post PCN was 7.5

months, but if patients developed ureteric obstruction while already on hormones, the mean survival decreased to 4.5 months. In the context of newly diagnosed and hormone-naïve patients, the survival increased to a mean of 16 months (range: 1–38 months) [23]. Similarly, Harris et al. found that survival was longer for the hormone-naïve group (226.5 days) when compared to 100.2 days in the castrate-resistant prostate cancer group [20].

In the context of bladder cancer, Ekici et al. looked at 23 patients with malignant ureteric obstruction due to bladder cancer, including patients with new diagnosis of locally advanced disease, disease recurrence post cystectomy, and those with metastatic disease. There was a mean survival of 4.9 months (range: 1–14 months). Eighteen (78%) died of disease progression or irreversible renal failure after malignant ureteric obstruction during the study period [17].

Romero et al. found that prognosis was worse in patients over 52 years old and in patients with bladder cancer or hormone refractory prostate cancer, rather than cervical cancer, but patient numbers were small ($n = 43$), so this may not be generalisable [18]. Misra et al. reported a median survival post PCN insertion as only 78 days (range: 4–1137 days) and also described that the subset of bladder cancer patients seemed to do more poorly [12]. In contradiction to these findings, Jalbani described an improved median survival in urogenital malignancies (bladder and prostate) of 350 days (range: 150–700 days) when compared to non-urogenital malignancies, except lymphoma (gynaecological, colorectal, breast, and gallbladder cancers) where the median survival was only 25 days (range: 7–80 days) [8].

Folkard et al. found that the average survival time post PCN was 139 days, and there was no significant difference between the cancer subgroups in terms of survival time post nephrostomy. They also showed that a greater improvement in renal function did not improve the survival time. A large proportion of their patients (65.7%) did not undergo further oncological treatment post PCN as they became too frail for it [25].

3.3.2. Prognostic Indicators

Alawneh et al. found that the factors associated with a shorter survival time were type of malignancy, bilateral hydronephrosis, serum albumin <3.5 mg/dL, presence of metastases, ascites, or pleural effusion. Survival was better if patients had only one risk factor, with median survival 17.6 months vs. 1.7 months if four risk factors were present. The overall 12-month survival in their paper was 33.7% [9]. Ishioka [15] found that the factors associated with a poorer prognosis included colorectal cancer, three or more events related to metastatic disease, degree of hydronephrosis, and serum albumin <3 g/dL.

Lienert et al.'s [10] prognostic indicators were consistent with previously discussed studies; a serum albumin <3 mg/dL and three or more events related to dissemination of cancer were factors significantly associated with shorter mean survival. Moreover, a sodium <135 mEq/L was found to be a significant prognostic factor. In this study, degree of hydronephrosis was not found to be a significant prognostic factor.

Nariculum et al. [23] showed that the mean survival for newly diagnosed patients (hormone-naïve) was 16 months (range: 1–38 months), compared to patients who developed ureteric obstruction while on hormones, where the mean survival was only 4.5 months (range: 10 days to 17 months). This was also shown by Harris et al., who showed that hormone-naïve patients survived longer at 226.5 days, compared to 114.3 days in hormone-responsive groups and 100.2 days in the hormone-resistant group. Another prognostic factor was the failure of renal function to improve despite nephrostomies, and if the post-procedure urea and creatinine went below 15 mmol/L and below 250 µmol/L, respectively, then the mean survival time was 192.4 days, but if the renal function did not improve, then the mean survival was only 30.7 days [20].

Romero et al. showed that the poor prognostic factors in their study were age above 52 years and patients with bladder and hormone refractory prostate cancer [18]. Misra also showed that patients with bladder cancer had a worse prognosis [12]. In contrast, Radecka et al. [3] and Jalbani et al. [8] showed an improved survival in patients with bladder cancer. De Souza et al. demonstrated that the finding of hypotension unrelated to septic symptoms was a risk factor for progression to death [24].

3.3.3. Complications of PCN

Nineteen studies commented on the complication rates (Table 2). The overall complication rate ranged from 7% to 87%. The majority of the complications were minor, including urinary tract infection, haematuria, skin infection, malposition/dislodgement of PCN tubing and self-limiting fever. There was, however, a reasonably high rate of kinking, dislodgement, or loss of nephrostomy requiring reinsertion. There were some major complications described, including two patients who required a nephrectomy due to severe infection and peri-renal abscesses [9].

Table 2. Complications of percutaneous nephrostomy (PCN) insertion.

Author	Type of Complication and %	Overall Complications
Ekici et al. [17]	Occlusion/dislodgement/malposition 30%	30%
Little et al. [26]	Occlusion/dislodgement/malposition 13%	13%
Tanaka et al. [16]	Infection/sepsis 54%	54%
Romero et al. [18]	Nephrectomy 5%	42%
Wilson et al. [19]	Occlusion/dislodgement/malposition 46.2%	46.2%
Carrafiello et al. [13]	Occlusion/dislodgement/malposition 17.3% Haematuria 1%	18.3%
Radecka et al. [3]	Occlusion/dislodgement/malposition 7%	7%
Aravantinos et al. [21]	Infection/sepsis 55% Transfusion 2.9%	47.9%
Dienstmann et al. [22]	Infection/sepsis 32% Occlusion/dislodgement/malposition 18% Death 4% Pain 2% Haematuria 2%	58%
Ishioka et al. [15]	Infection/sepsis 13% Occlusion/dislodgement/malposition 19% Haematuria 8%	40%
Nariculam et al. [23]	Infection/sepsis 4% Occlusion/dislodgement/malposition 12% Haematuria 8%	24%
Lienert et al. [10]	Infection/sepsis 22.4% Occlusion/dislodgement/malposition 63% Haematuria 2%	87%
Jalbani et al. [8]	Infection/sepsis 7.5% Occlusion/dislodgement/malposition 37.5% Haematuria 5%	50%
Plesinac-Karapandzic et al. [11]	Infection/sepsis 39.2% Occlusion/dislodgement/malposition 37.6%	76.8%
Malik et al. [14]	-	4–25%
Misra et al. [12]	-	27%
De Souza et al. [24]	Infection/sepsis 42% Occlusion/dislodgement/malposition 15.5% Perirenal haematoma <5%	62.5%
McDevitt et al. [6]	Infection/sepsis 24% Occlusion/dislodgement/malposition 42.5%	66.5%
Folkard et al. [25]	-	39%

McDevitt et al. specifically looked at the number of routine vs. emergency PCN changes. Out of 87 PCN exchanges or reinsertions, only 33% were routine and 67% were for emergency reasons such as infection, obstruction, displacement, or mechanical complications [6].

Insertion of the initial PCN has good rates of technical success. Aravantinos et al. reported a 2.5% failure rate, with no serious complications, a minor temperature rise of 55%, and a transfusion rate of 2.9%; however, they commented on pre-existing anaemia, and therefore this may not be related to the PCN insertion itself. They also reported that a small proportion of patients (4.4%) needed staged a second nephrostomy tube due to persistent uraemia despite a unilateral nephrostomy tube [21].

3.3.4. Bilateral vs. Unilateral PCN

One point of interest was whether in order to improve QoL in patients with bilateral hydronephrosis secondary to malignant ureteric obstruction, a unilateral nephrostomy was sufficient. Thirteen studies commented on whether they inserted unilateral or bilateral nephrostomies. In prostate cancer, one study reported that the mean survival for unilateral nephrostomy patients was better (157.6 days) than for those who required bilateral nephrostomies, whether they were placed simultaneously or staged [20]. This could be due to the fact that they also demonstrated that a worse prognosis is linked with bilateral hydronephrosis. In one study of mixed malignancies, 92% of the patients had bilateral hydronephrosis and their aim was to trial unilateral PCN. Only 4.4% patients required a second-stage nephrostomy due to persistent uraemia despite having a unilateral nephrostomy [21].

3.3.5. Quality of Life after PCN

There are no validated questionnaires specifically looking at QoL with nephrostomies in cancer patients [27]. A wide range of methods for determining quality of life with a nephrostomy were used throughout the studies. Aravantinos et al. [21] used the QoL questionnaire EORTC-QLC-C30 [28] and found that QoL improved at 1 month, and of the different cancer subgroups, it was better in the prostate cancer subgroup. Wilson et al. used the criteria of Grabstald and McPhee to define 'useful quality of life' and found 17/32 (53.1%) did not fulfil such criteria, and the subgroup of bladder cancer patients had poorer outcomes [19]. Misra used the Watkinson criterion (if the patient was able to leave hospital for 6 weeks or more), finding that 64% would have satisfied this criterion [12]. In the studies that measured QoL, only around half of the patients achieved an adequate QoL post PCN insertion.

3.3.6. In-Hospital Stay after PCN

The time spent in hospital following PCN insertion was highly variable and poorly reported (Table 1). Romero found that the percentage of lifetime left that was spent in hospital was 17.7%, and 57.7% of those discharged from hospital had to be readmitted (either due to disease progression or complications from PCN) [18]. Wilson reported a mean hospital stay of 29 days from PCN insertion to death or end of study period, and each patient was readmitted an average of 1.6 times until death [19]. Misra reported a median hospital stay post PCN of 23 days (range: 3–89), with 29% of a patient's end of life spent in hospital [12]. Folkard had a mean hospital stay of 14 days post PCN; however, 39% of the patients were readmitted, and 20% spent their remaining life in hospital [25].

Many patients with advanced malignancies die in hospital despite PCN insertion, and nine studies reported the percentage of patients who died on the same hospital admission as their PCN was placed [8,12,16,18–20,22,24,25]. The mean percentage of patients who died on the same hospital admission as their PCN insertion was 30.8% and ranged from 12.5% to 70% (Figure 2).

4. Discussion

4.1. Findings of Our Study

The mean survival time varied from 2.6 to 8.5 months post initial PCN insertion across the studies, with an average survival time of 5.9 months (Figure 2, Table 1). The majority of studies agreed that hormone-naïve prostate cancer had a longer survival time post PCN insertion, whereas bladder cancer, cervical cancer, and hormone refractory prostate cancer all had shortened life expectancies. Poor prognostic indicators throughout the studies were patients who had already undergone cancer treatment, presence of multiple metastasis, type of cancer, degree of hydronephrosis, and a low serum albumin concentration. The number of days spent in hospital post PCN insertion were high (Table 1) and a third of the patients (range: 12.5–70%) died on the same admission while they were admitted to hospital (Figure 2).

4.2. Patient Counselling

The ethics of palliative urinary decompression have been debated, and many factors must be taken into account, such as the type and stage of malignancy, the ability for further palliative treatment, patient's quality and quantity of life along with their preference. Malignant ureteric obstruction from pelvic malignancies often presents a significant treatment dilemma for urologists. While PCN insertion is relatively safe, patients with advanced malignancies tend to have a higher risk of PCN-related complications (Table 2) and spend a large proportion of their time in hospitals. PCNs should only be pursued after thoughtful counselling regarding further treatment options and likely disease prognosis.

4.3. Quality of Life

There are no validated questionnaires specifically looking at QoL with nephrostomies in cancer patients [27]. A wide range of methods for determining QoL with a nephrostomy were used throughout the studies, ranging from whether the patient ever left hospital at all, to whether they left hospital for 6 weeks or more (Watkinson criteria [29]), to scoring them on four criteria; of little or no pain, full mental capacity, few complications related to PCN insertion, and the ability to return home (Grabstald and McPhee criteria [19]), to using EORTC-QLC-C30 questionnaires [28]. It is difficult to ascertain whether QoL is worse after PCN insertion due to the procedure, or the progression of the cancer; hence a standardised questionnaire would be useful in ascertaining this and could aid patients in making the decision on whether or not to proceed with a nephrostomy [27].

4.4. Costs of Replacement of PCN

McDevitt et al. looked at patients who had nephrostomies placed for malignant ureteric obstruction, and the causes of PCN exchanges during the follow-up period. There were 87 exchanges performed, and of those, 29/87 (33.3%) were routine elective changes, but 58/87 (66.7%) were unplanned and due to complications, such as infection (21/87, 33%), obstruction (23/87, 26%) or mechanical complications (14/87, 16%). The cost of emergency exchange vs. routine exchange was modelled to be higher, and they therefore hypothesised that decreasing the length of time to routine exchange from 90 days to 60 days would decrease the amount of readmissions for emergency exchange or replacement, which would decrease the overall cost [6].

4.5. Conversion of PCN to Ureteric Stents

In some cases, where PCN has been inserted primarily, it may be possible to convert it to an indwelling ureteric stent, usually via antegrade stenting. Wilson and colleagues reported that in 34.4% of cases, they were able to have PCN converted to an indwelling stent [19], and Misra et al. reported that 56% of all PCNs were subsequently antegradely stented and rendered nephrostomy free [12]. Folkard reported that 65% of PCNs were converted to stents.

4.6. Limitations

Almost all of the studies were retrospective, and with historic data, which made it difficult to apply them to today's cancer patients with recent advances in cancer treatment. These studies cover a heterogeneous population with some having a variety of different primary cancers, while others focus on a single cancer type, which makes interpretation difficult. As novel immunotherapy and chemotherapy options emerge, the ability to predict prognosis is more guarded, and newer information is needed to aid decision making. There were no data from situations where patients presented with hydronephrosis and the decision was not to perform PCN, and how their QoL and length of life compared to those with PCN.

Since the studies reported included a wide time interval (from 2003 to 2020), it should be appropriate to take into account that some malignancies have improved treatment options with potential benefits to prognosis and quality of life. For example, in colorectal cancer, starting from 2004 several drugs have been introduced (cetuximab, bevacizumab, and panitumumab) with advantage on cancer-specific survival. Similar improvements have been reported in prostate cancer from 2011 with new hormone-based therapies (abiraterone and enzalutamide) in metastatic castration-resistant patients, and from 2015 in metastatic hormone-sensitive patients. This treatment may also affect the quality of life and the number of days spent in hospital. Moreover, in selected cases, the option of a new treatment line can justify the insertion of ureteric stent or nephrostomy.

The retrospective nature of the included papers with different inclusion criteria makes it liable to selection bias and hence difficult to draw meaningful comparisons. Given that almost a third of the patients died on the same hospital admission as their PCN insertion suggests that a high number of reported PCNs were performed for palliative reasons. The decision on nephrostomy would have to be individualised for a given patient and must take into account their medical condition and underlying disease status.

4.7. Areas of Future Research

Prognosis of patients with malignant ureteric obstruction is mostly dependent on further treatment strategies. In recent years, there has been a big leap in oncological therapies, many of which are reliant on good renal function. In many situations now, where there is malignant ureteric obstruction, a patient may still have further options for palliative chemotherapy, immunotherapy or novel hormone therapies. However, if there are no options in reserve, the prognosis is poor with or without nephrostomies, and end-of-life care should be discussed with the patient and relatives, rather than proceeding with invasive interventions that have no impact on disease progression. Complications and death due to locally invasive cancer should be weighed against complications and death due to uraemia.

5. Conclusions

There is little doubt about the benefits of percutaneous nephrostomy for patients with a new diagnosis of disease, allowing improvement of renal function to allow staging investigations. However, in patients in the end stages of their cancer, PCN insertion should only be placed after thoughtful counselling regarding further treatment options available and disease prognosis, given that with advanced malignancies, many patients have a short life expectancy, spending most of their time in the hospital with a poor quality of life.

Author Contributions: Conceptualization, B.K.S.; methodology, B.K.S., F.J.N., S.J.D.; formal analysis, F.J.N., S.J.D.; data curation, F.J.N., S.J.D.; writing—original draft preparation, S.J.D., F.J.N.; writing—review and editing, F.J.N., B.K.S.; supervision, B.K.S.; All authors have read and agreed to the published version of the manuscript.

Funding: This research received no external funding.

Institutional Review Board Statement: Not applicable.

Informed Consent Statement: Not applicable.

Conflicts of Interest: The authors declare no conflict of interests.

References

1. Bigum, L.H.; Spielmann, M.E.; Juhl, G.; Rasmussen, A. A qualitative study exploring male cancer patients' experiences with percutaneous nephrostomy. *Scand. J. Urol.* **2014**, *49*, 162–168. [CrossRef]
2. Kouba, E.; Wallen, E.M.; Pruthi, R.J. Management of ureteral obstruction due to advanced malignancy: Optimising therapeutic and palliative outcomes. *J. Urol.* **2008**, *180*, 444–450. [CrossRef]
3. Radecka, E.; Magnusson, A. Complications associated with percutaneous nephrostomies. A retrospective study. *Acta Radiol.* **2004**, *45*, 184–188. [CrossRef]
4. Wah, T.M.; Weston, M.J.; Irving, H.C. Percutaneous nephrostomy insertion: Outcome data from a prospective multi-operator sudy at a UK training centre. *Clin. Radiol.* **2004**, *59*, 255–261. [CrossRef]
5. Patel, U.; Hussain, F.F. Percutaneous Nephrostomy of Nondilated Renal Collecting Systems with Fluoroscopic Guidance: Technique and Results. *Radiology* **2004**, *233*, 226–233. [CrossRef] [PubMed]
6. McDevitt, J.L.; Acosta-Torres, S.; Zhang, N.; Hu, T.; Odu, A.; Wang, J.; Xi, Y.; Lamus, D.; Miller, D.S.; Pillai, A.K. Long-Term Percutaneous Nephrostomy Management of Malignant Urinary Obstruction: Estimation of Optimal Exchange Frequency and Estimation of the Financial Impact of Patient Compliance. *J. Vasc. Interv. Radiol.* **2017**, *28*, 1036–1042.e8. [CrossRef] [PubMed]
7. Liberati, A.; Altman, D.G.; Tetzlaff, J.; Mulrow, C.; Gøtzsche, P.C.; Ioannidis, J.P.A.; Clarke, M.; Devereaux, P.J.; Kleijnen, J.; Moher, D. The PRISMA statement for reporting systematic reviews and meta-analyses of studies that evaluate healthcare interventions: Explanation and elaboration. *BMJ* **2009**, *339*, b2700. [CrossRef] [PubMed]
8. Jalbani, M.H.; Deenari, R.A.; Dholia, K.R.; Oad, A.K.; Arbani, I.A. Role of percutaneous nephrostomy (PCN) in malignant ureteral obstruction. *J. Pak. Med. Assoc.* **2010**, *60*, 280–283.
9. Alawneh, A.; Tuqan, W.; Innabi, A.; Al-Nimer, Y.; Azzouqah, O.; Rimawi, D.; Taqash, A.; Elkhatib, M.; Klepstad, P. Clinical Factors Associated With a Short Survival Time After Percutaneous Nephrostomy for Ureteric Obstruction in Cancer Patients: An Updated Model. *J. Pain Symptom Manag.* **2016**, *51*, 255–261. [CrossRef]
10. Lienert, A.; Ing, A.; Mark, S. Prognostic factors in malignant ureteric obstruction. *BJU Int.* **2009**, *104*, 938–941. [CrossRef]
11. Plesinac-Karapandzic, V.; Masulovic, D.; Markovic, B.; Djuric-Stefanovic, A.; Plesinac, S.; Vucicevic, D.; Milovanovic, Z.; Milosevic, Z. Percutaneous nephrostomy in the management of advanced and terminal-stage gynecologic malignancies: Outcome and complications. *Eur. J. Gynaecol. Oncol.* **2010**, *31*, 645–650.
12. Misra, S.; Coker, C.; Richenberg, J. Percutaneous nephrostomy for ureteric obstruction due to advanced pelvic malignancy: Have we got the balance right yet? *Int. Urol. Nephrol.* **2013**, *45*, 627–632. [CrossRef]
13. Carrafiello, G.; Laganà, D.; Mangini, M.; Lumia, D.; Recaldini, C.; Bacuzzi, A.; Marconi, A.; Mira, A.; Cuffari, S.; Fugazzola, C. Complications of percutaneous nephrostomy in the treatment of malignant ureteral obstructions: Single–centre review. *La Radiol. Med.* **2006**, *111*, 562–571. [CrossRef]
14. Malik, M.A.; Mahmood, T.; Khan, J.H.; Hanif, A.; Bajwa, I.A. Experience of percutaneous nephrostomy (PCN) in advanced ca prostate. *PJMHS* **2010**, *4*, 537–541.
15. Ishioka, J.; Kzgeyama, Y.; Inoue, M.; Higashi, Y.; Kihara, K. Prognostic Model for predicting survival after palliative urinary diversion for utereral obstruction: Analysis of 140 cases. *J. Urol.* **2008**, *180*, 618–621. [CrossRef]
16. Tanaka, T.; Yanase, M.; Takatsuka, K. Clinical course in patients with percutaneous nephrostomy for hydronephrosis associated with advanced cancer. *Hinyokika Kiyo. Acta Urol. Jpn.* **2004**, *50*, 457–462.
17. Ekici, S.; Şahin, A.; Özen, H. Percutaneous Nephrostomy in the Management of Malignant Ureteral Obstruction Secondary to Bladder Cancer. *J. Endourol.* **2001**, *15*, 827–829. [CrossRef]
18. Romero, F.R.; Broglio, M.; Pires, S.R.; Roca, R.F.; Guibu, I.A.; Perez, M.D. Indications for percutaneous nephrostomy in patients with obstructive uropathy due to malignant Urogenital neoplasias. *Int. Braz. J. Urol.* **2005**, *31*, 117–124. [CrossRef] [PubMed]
19. Wilson, J.R.; Urwin, G.H.; Stower, M.J. The role of percutaneous nephrostomy in malignant ureteric obstruction. *Ann. R. Coll. Surg. Engl.* **2005**, *87*, 21–24. [CrossRef] [PubMed]
20. Harris, M.R.E.; Speakman, M.J. Nephrostomies in obstructive uropathy; how should hormone resistant prostate cancer patients be managed and can we predict who will benefit? *Prostate Cancer Prostatic Dis.* **2006**, *9*, 42–44. [CrossRef]
21. Aravantinos, E.; Anagnostou, T.; Karatzas, A.D.; Papakonstantinou, W.; Samarinas, M.; Melekos, M.D. Percutaneous nephrostomy in patients with tumors of advanced stage: Treatment dilemmas and impact on clinical course and Qaulity of life. *J. Endourol.* **2007**, *21*, 1297–1302. [CrossRef]
22. Dienstmann, R.; Pinto, C.D.S.; Pereira, M.T.; Small, I.Á.; Gil Ferreira, C. Palliative Percutaneous Nephrostomy in Recurrent Cervical Cancer: A Retrospective Analysis of 50 Consecutive Cases. *J. Pain Symptom Manag.* **2008**, *36*, 185–190. [CrossRef] [PubMed]
23. Nariculam, J.; Murphy, D.G.; Jenner, C.; Sellars, N.; Gwyther, S.; Gordon, S.G.; Swinn, M.J. Nephrostomy insertion for patients with bilateral ureteric obstruction caused by prostate cancer. *Br. J. Radiol.* **2009**, *82*, 571–576. [CrossRef]
24. De Souza, A.C.P.; Souza, A.N.; Kirsztajn, R.; Kirsztajn, G.M. Cervical cancer: Renal Complications and survival after percutaneous nephrostomy. *Rev. Assoc. Med. Bras.* **2016**, *62*, 255–261. [CrossRef] [PubMed]

25. Folkard, S.S.; Banerjee, S.; Menzies-Wilson, R.; Reason, J.; Psallidas, E.; Clissold, E.; Al-Mushatat, A.; Chaudhri, S.; Green, J.S.A. Percutaneous nephrostomy in obstructing pelvic malignancy does not facilitate further oncological treatment. *Int. Urol. Nephrol.* **2020**, *52*, 1625–1628. [CrossRef]
26. Little, B.; Ho, K.J.; Gawley, S.; Young, M. Use of nephrostomy tubes in ureteric obstruction from incurable malignancy. *Int. J. Clin. Pract.* **2003**, *57*, 180–181. [PubMed]
27. New, F.; Deverill, S.; Somani, B.K. Role of percutaneous nephrostomy in end of life prostate cancer patients: A systematic review of the literature. *Cent. Eur. J. Urol.* **2018**, *71*, 404–409. [CrossRef]
28. Aaronson, N.K.; Ahmedzai, S.; Bergman, B.; Bullinger, M.; Cull, A.; Duez, N.J.; Filiberti, A.; Flechtner, H.; Fleishman, S.B.; De Haes, J.C.; et al. The European Organization for Research and Treatment of Cancer QLQ-C30: A Quality-of-Life Instrument for Use in International Clinical Trials in Oncology. *J. Natl. Cancer Inst.* **1993**, *85*, 365–376. [CrossRef]
29. Watkinson, A.; A'Hern, R.; Jones, A.; King, D.; Moskovic, E. The role of percutaneous nephrostomy in malignant urinary tract obstruction. *Clin. Radiol.* **1993**, *47*, 32–35. [CrossRef]

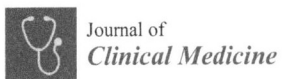

Review

Artificial Intelligence and Its Impact on Urological Diseases and Management: A Comprehensive Review of the Literature

B. M. Zeeshan Hameed [1,2,3,4], Aiswarya V. L. S. Dhavileswarapu [5], Syed Zahid Raza [6], Hadis Karimi [7], Harneet Singh Khanuja [8], Dasharathraj K. Shetty [9], Sufyan Ibrahim [3,10], Milap J. Shah [1,3], Nithesh Naik [3,4,11,*], Rahul Paul [12], Bhavan Prasad Rai [13] and Bhaskar K. Somani [1,3,14]

1. Department of Urology, Kasturba Medical College Manipal, Manipal Academy of Higher Education, Manipal 576104, Karnataka, India; zeeshanhameedbm@gmail.com (B.M.Z.H.); drmilapshah@gmail.com (M.J.S.); bhaskarsomani@yahoo.com (B.K.S.)
2. KMC Innovation Centre, Manipal Academy of Higher Education, Manipal 576104, Karnataka, India
3. iTRUE (International Training and Research in Uro-Oncology and Endourology) Group, Manipal 576104, Karnataka, India; sufyan.ibrahim2@gmail.com
4. Curiouz Techlab Private Limited, Manipal Government of Karnataka Bioincubator, Manipal 576104, Karnataka, India
5. Department of Electronics and Communication, GITAM University, Gandhi Nagar, Rushi Konda, Visakhapatnam 530045, Andhra Pradesh, India; aash.dhavil@gmail.com
6. Department of Urology, Dr. B.R. Ambedkar Medical College, Bengaluru 560045, Karnataka, India; syed.zahid.raza@gmail.com
7. Manipal College of Pharmaceutical Sciences, Manipal Academy of Higher Education, Manipal 576104, Karnataka, India; hadiskarimi1997@gmail.com
8. Department of Information and Communication Technology, Manipal Institute of Technology, Manipal Academy of Higher Education, Manipal 576104, Karnataka, India; hskhanuja2@gmail.com
9. Department of Humanities and Management, Manipal Institute of Technology, Manipal Academy of Higher Education, Manipal 576104, Karnataka, India; raja.shetty@manipal.edu
10. Kasturba Medical College Manipal, Manipal Academy of Higher Education, Manipal 576104, Karnataka, India
11. Department of Mechanical and Manufacturing, Manipal Institute of Technology, Manipal Academy of Higher Education, Manipal 576104, Karnataka, India
12. Department of Radiation Oncology, Massachusetts General Hospital, Harvard Medical School, Boston, MA 02115, USA; rpaul7@mgh.harvard.edu
13. Department of Urology, Freeman Hospital, Newcastle NE7 7DN, UK; urobhavan@gmail.com
14. Department of Urology, University Hospital Southampton NHS Trust, Southampton SO16 6YD, UK
* Correspondence: nithesh.naik@manipal.edu

Abstract: Recent advances in artificial intelligence (AI) have certainly had a significant impact on the healthcare industry. In urology, AI has been widely adopted to deal with numerous disorders, irrespective of their severity, extending from conditions such as benign prostate hyperplasia to critical illnesses such as urothelial and prostate cancer. In this article, we aim to discuss how algorithms and techniques of artificial intelligence are equipped in the field of urology to detect, treat, and estimate the outcomes of urological diseases. Furthermore, we explain the advantages that come from using AI over any existing traditional methods.

Keywords: urology; artificial intelligence; machine learning; urinary incontinence; kidney stone disease; fertility; reproductive urology; renal cell carcinoma; hydronephrosis; urinary reflux; urolithiasis; endourology; pediatric urology; prostate cancer; bladder cancer

1. Introduction

Advances made in digital technologies, electronic health records, and computing power are producing vast amounts of data in the medical field [1]. With expanded channels, quantity, and quality of data, physicians encounter new obstacles while performing data analysis to establish a reliable diagnosis, planning individualized care, and forecasting the future. Thus, physicians are now relying on artificial intelligence (AI) to build automated models to enhance patient treatment across all aspects of healthcare [2].

In the healthcare industry, AI refers to all the applications, systems, algorithms, and devices that help physicians in providing healthcare based on computer systems and big data. Medical data are ideally used for advising doctors and patients during the decision-making process and identifying the most suitable treatment. The role of AI here is to create new methods for analyzing labor-intensive data, which involves the usage of disciplines of AI. Along with providing improved patient care, it will also enhance efficiency and research and development (R&D), in addition to highlighting disease patterns and correlations earlier than what would be possible via traditional methods. In recent times, AI has seen an explosion in investment and application in the field of medicine, as there is cumulative evidence that it may enhance the delivery of healthcare [3]. This article discusses how AI algorithms and techniques are used in the medical field to detect, treat, and estimate the outcomes of urological diseases and further explains the advantages of using AI over any existing methods.

2. Materials and Methods

2.1. Search Strategy and Article Selection

A non-systematic review of the literature associated with urology and artificial intelligence that was published between the years 2010 and 2020 was conducted in October 2020 using PubMed and MEDLINE, along with Scopus and Google Scholar. The search strategy involved using a search string based on a set of keywords that included the following: urology, artificial intelligence, machine learning, urinary incontinence, kidney stone disease, fertility, reproductive urology, renal cell carcinoma, hydronephrosis, urinary reflux, urolithiasis, endourology, pediatric urology, prostate cancer, and bladder cancer.

Inclusion criteria:
1. Articles related to artificial intelligence in urology;
2. Original articles of full-text length covering the diagnoses, treatment plans, and results of urologic conditions.

Exclusion criteria:
1. Abstracts, review articles, and chapters from books;
2. Animal, laboratory, or cadaveric studies.

The review of the literature was performed in compliance with the guidelines for inclusion and exclusion criteria. The assessment of titles and abstracts followed by the screening and assessment of the full article text was done according to the inclusion criteria for the selected articles. Further, a manual review of the references list for the chosen articles was conducted to screen for any supplementary work of interest. After a discussion, our authors successfully resolved the disagreements regarding the eligibility for a consensus decision.

2.2. What Is Artificial Intelligence?

AI emphasizes constructing an autonomous computer that will effectively execute activities done by humans, using sophisticated non-linear mathematical simulation systems with simple building blocks that replicate human neurons. It begins by searching for ways in which a human mind perceives, understands, and executes cognitive functions. The human mind is capable of intelligence, creativity, language recognition, memory, pattern identification, vision, reasoning, and the creation of ties among facts. AI aims to replicate the aforementioned skills to perform wide-ranging functions, from small, manageable tasks like object recognition to complex tasks like forecasting. AI strategies include learning from known data without bias, dependent only on statistical models, and estimating unknown data about the future, thereby making the task of decision-making smarter and easier [2].

The ultimate goal of AI is to build a machine that can perceive its environment and perform tasks to maximize its probability of success. The process of achieving this goal is quite complex and involves various AI subfields such as machine learning (ML), artificial neural networks (ANNs) and deep learning (DL), natural language processing (NLP), computer vision, predictive analytics, evolutionary and genetic computing, expert systems, vision recognition, and speech processing, of which most are used in medicine and healthcare today. Thus, some of them need defining for further discussion on the clinical impact of artificial intelligence on various sub-specialties of urology. Figure 1 shows the relationship between artificial intelligence (AI), machine learning (ML), and deep learning (DL).

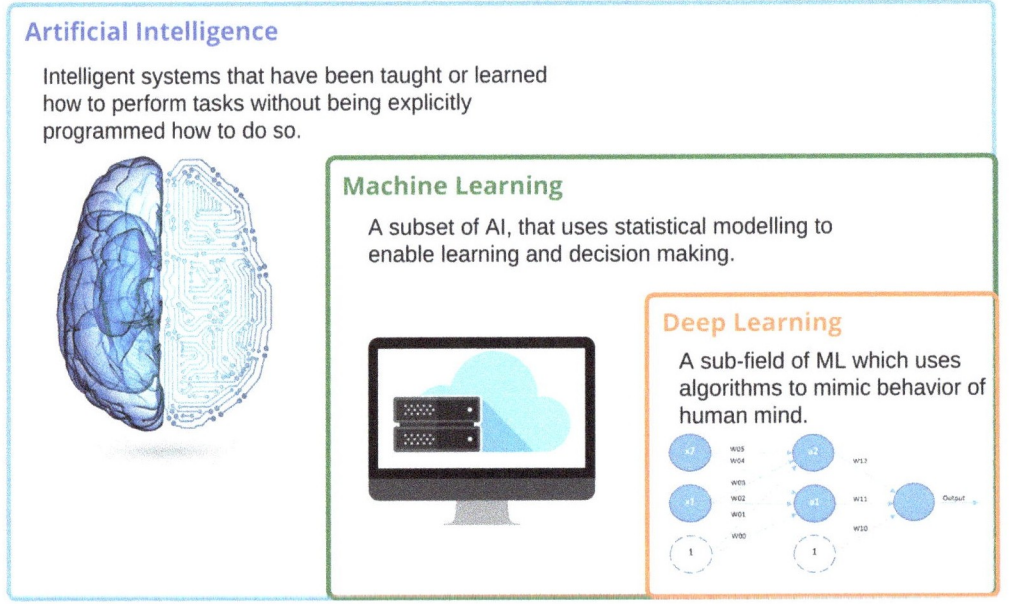

Figure 1. The relationship between artificial intelligence (AI), machine learning (ML), and deep learning (DL).

Machine learning is the process of teaching a computer to make accurate predictions with the help of algorithms that are trained and made to learn from past experiences in a model that maps features to the corresponding outcome variables. The primary aim of ML is to allow the computer to automatically learn when data are fed. An artificial neural network is the basis of deep learning and a subfield of machine learning. ANNs are defined as highly structured information processing units that, along with their synaptic strengths, called weights, mimic the computational abilities of the human brain and nervous system. The neurons are arranged in a series of layers where the weights are modified gradually during the learning process to yield minimum to no error in the input–output mapping. A neural network that has a significant number of layers is called a deep learning network. Being a subfield that holds paramount importance in AI, neural networks have naturally found promising applications in medicine and healthcare, including cardiology, electromyography, electroencephalography, therapeutic drug monitoring for patient care, and sleep apnea.

Decision trees are one of the predictive modeling approaches used in ML, constructed in an algorithmic approach to identifying ways of splitting the dataset based on different conditions. A simple way to describe a decision tree's working would be to assume a decision node with two or more possible choices. A random forest is an algorithm built with a large number of decision trees that operate as an ensemble. These algorithms are widely adopted in the healthcare industry to determine the patient's most favorable choice, such as telehealth services.

Another AI subfield that plays a critical role in healthcare is natural language processing, which is concerned with the interaction between the computer and human languages. The biggest challenge in clinical research is to deal with data that are lacking in volume or detail, which is a result of data previously being recorded in narrative clinical documentation. Some of AI's most promising uses in healthcare include predictive analytics, precision medicine, diagnostic imaging of diseases, and clinical decision support.

2.3. Applications of AI in Urology

Urology is a field that rapidly expanded through the history of medicine and is continually growing by adopting newer technology to achieve better patient outcomes [4]. Urology being a healthcare segment that deals mainly with male and female urinary tracts and male reproductive organs, the underlying diseases and conditions in these specific areas could become severe if not addressed earlier. Figure 2 shows the role of artificial intelligence in urology.

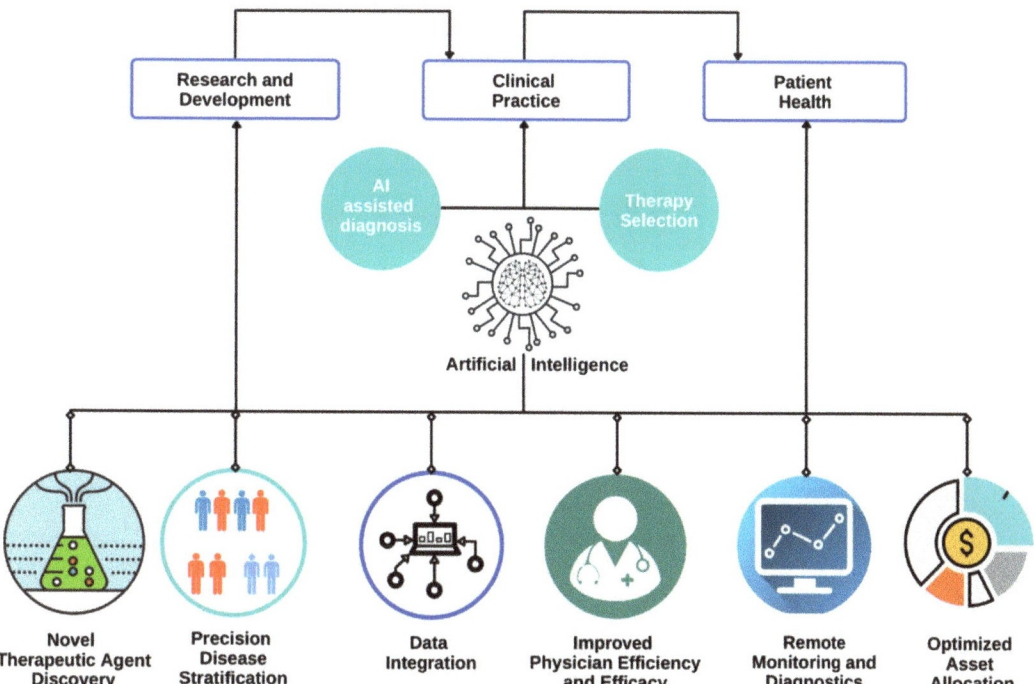

Figure 2. Role of artificial intelligence in urology.

AI has been widely adopted in the field for early diagnosis, for providing an effective treatment plan, and in surgical specialties. AI is playing an important role and helping physicians in decision making for patients with urological disorders (Figure 3). In the past 5 years, there has been an emergence of studies affirming the safe and effective augmented-reality (AR) experiences in urology. Modern urologists are using a robotic arm with seven degrees of freedom to remove the kidney remotely, using augmented reality with image overlay [5]. AR is significantly improving the integration of information into the surgical workflow, making minimally invasive procedures less complicated for surgeons. It is bringing innovative approaches in medical education as well as surgical interventions, aiding richer and more interactive experiences. Similarly, there are other technologies combined with AI that impact the field to a great extent. Within urology, there are several sub-specialties, among which urologic oncology, reproductive urology, renal transplant, and pediatric urology are some specialties that have leveraged AI to provide better patient care through developments in diagnostics, treatment planning, and surgical skill assessment [5]. The application of AI in these subfields is discussed below.

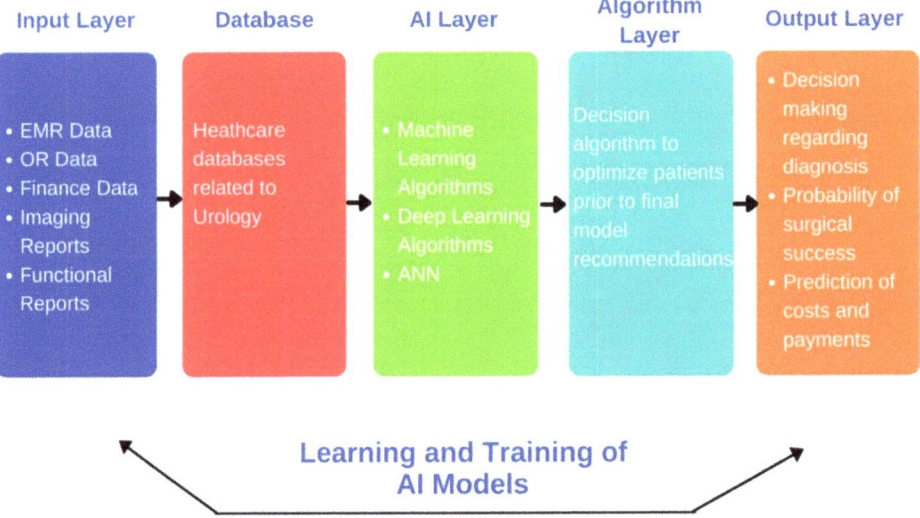

Figure 3. Artificial intelligence in decision making in patients with urological disorders.

3. Diagnosis

3.1. Urologic Oncology

It is a sub-specialty of urology that is associated with the diagnosis and treatment of cancers in the urinary tract of the human body and male reproductive organs. Urological cancers are relatively common, with prostate, bladder, and kidney cancers among the 10 most prevalent cancers diagnosed in the United States.

3.2. Prostate Cancer

The data that are widely used for developing AI algorithms are clinicopathological data of patients abstracted from their electronic medical records (EMRs) because of their high evaluability. With clinical data from 944 Korean patients for predicting organ-confined prostate cancer and non-organ-confined disease, Kim et al. [6] developed a set of ML applications (Table 1). In comparison, Partin tables achieved an accuracy of 66% when using the same dataset. This study highlighted that one can achieve better forecasting results using ML algorithms than using standard statistical models.

Researchers have suggested methods of using AI to simplify the diagnosis and classification of prostate cancer, which has become possible due to the advances in medical imaging and the evidence surrounding it. Using various radiomic features from multiparametric MRI (Magnetic resonance imaging), AI applications have been equipped for detecting prostate cancer [7,8] or for estimating multiparametric MRI Gleason scores [9,10] (Table 1). What also makes AI better than traditional diagnostic standards is its ability to get trained by and learn from complex, multi-variable, big data, thereby improving over time. The ML models displayed an average performance increase of 33–80% for MRI-negative biopsy-positive and 30–60% for MRI-positive biopsy-negative patients when developed using Prostate Imaging Reporting and Data Systems. Fehr et al. [10] observed that ML algorithms had an advantage over unimodal classifiers as they performed more effectively in both identifying the disease and forecasting the correct Gleason score.

Table 1. Studies using AI to diagnose prostate cancer.

Study	Application of the Study	Type of Study	Size of the Sample Used	Features Used for Training	Algorithms Used	Accuracy, %	Sensitivity, %	Specificity, %	AUC
Kim et al., 2017 [6]	Forecast of extracapsular expansion	Retrospective	944 patients (621 and 323 organ-confined disease and non-organ-confined disease, respectively)	PSA, Gleason score, clinical T stage, and positive prostate biopsy core count	NN	73.4	-	-	-
					SVM	75.0	-	-	-
					NB	74.8	-	-	-
					BNs	74.4	-	-	-
					CART	70.7	-	-	-
					RF	68.8	-	-	-
Algohary et al., 2018 [7]	Diagnosis based on MRI	Retrospective	56 patients	Radiomic MRI features chosen by unsupervised hierarchical clustering	QDA	72.0	75.0	60.0	-
					RF	32.0	42.0	30.0	-
					SVM	52.0	60.0	40.0	-
Ginsburg et al., 2017 [8]	Diagnosis based on MRI	Retrospective	80 patients	Radiomic MRI characteristics	LR	-	-	-	0.61–0.71
Fehr et al., 2015 [10]	Forecast of Gleason score using MRI	Retrospective	356 regions of interest from 147 patients	Radiomic MRI characteristics	t-Test SVM (Gleason 6 vs. ≥7)	73–83	-	-	0.83–0.90
					AdaBoost (Gleason 6 vs. ≥7)	64–73	-	-	0.60–0.74
					RFE-SVM (Gleason 6 vs. ≥7)	83–93	-	-	0.91–0.99
					t-Test SVM (Gleason 3 + 4 vs. 4 + 3)	66–81	-	-	0.94–0.99
					AdaBoost (Gleason 3 + 4 vs. 4 + 3)	73–79	-	-	0.75–0.80
					RFE-SVM (Gleason 3 + 4 vs. 4 + 3)	83–92	-	-	0.77–0.81
Kwak et al., 2017 [11]	Diagnosis based on images of tissue samples	Retrospective	653 tissue samples	HE-stained digitized images of the prostate specimen	Multiview boosting classifier (differentiate benign and malignant tissue)	-	-	-	0.98
					Multiview boosting classifier (differentiate epithelium and stroma)	-	-	-	0.97–0.99
Kwak et al., 2017 [12]	Diagnosis based on images of tissue samples	Retrospective	827 tissue samples	HE-stained digitized images of the prostate specimen	CNN	-	-	-	0.97
Nguyen et al., 2017 [13]	Estimation of Gleason score based on tissue samples from the prostate	Retrospective	368 prostate tissue samples (1 per patient)	HE-stained digitized images of the prostate specimen	RF (benign vs. malignant)	-	-	-	0.97 / 0.82
					LR (Gleason scoring 3 vs. 4)	-	-	-	0.82

Area Under the ROC Curve (AUC); Neural Network (NN); Support Vector Machine (SVM); Prostate Specific Antigen (PSA); Naive Bayes (NB); Bayesian Networks (BNs); Classification and Regression Tree (CART); Random Forest (RF); Quadratic Discriminant Analysis (QDA); Magnetic resonance imaging (MRI); Logistic Regression (LR); Recursive Feature Elimination (RFE); Hematoxylin and Eosin (HE).

Prostate cancer diagnosis depends on the pathologists reviewing specimen slides as well as assessing the same using Gleason scoring, and while the entire procedure takes a lot of time, it can cause intra-observer bias, depending on the experience of the pathologists. AI-assisted image analysis in clinical pathology combines automated image recognition, examination, as well as evaluation of digitalized tissue specimen images, allowing automatic and standardized pathology diagnosis (Table 1). Kwak et al. [11] developed an AI application for detecting the disease in optical pathology images of varying resolutions. The algorithm was able to achieve an accuracy of >97% on the same using segmented prostate specimen images. The aforementioned group also developed ANNs with the nuclear morphology of prostatic epithelial cells for the detection of cancer [12]. They were able to achieve an AUC (Area under the ROC Curve) score of 0.97 for the diagnosis of prostate cancer, surpassing diagnostic methods using handcrafted nuclear engineering technologies. Nguyen et al. [13] developed an ML algorithm to classify the Gleason score of prostate cancer. The classifier has different AUC scores when considering cancer and non-cancer specimens in distinguishing between epithelial tissue and stromal tissue, specifically 0.97 for the former and 0.87 for the latter. In addition, when provided five characteristics of histology, the algorithm achieved an AUC of 0.82 in distinguishing Gleason 3 vs. 4 cancer [13].

3.3. Urothelial Cancer

Bladder cancers, also known as urothelial carcinomas, begin in the cell lining of the bladder (i.e., non-muscle-invasive bladder cancer) and can spread to the muscle wall and beyond, to other tissues (i.e., muscle invasive or metastatic bladder cancer). They are highly curable when detected and treated early. Similar to prostate cancer, radiomic imaging and urinary metabolite markers have been used to diagnose urothelial cancer using AI techniques (Table 2). Xu et al. [14] developed ML algorithms with radiomic mpMRI characteristics for distinguishing between bladder tumor and normal bladder wall. Garapati et al. [15] used morphological and textural features of CT (Computed Tomography) urography for determining the stage of bladder cancer. The algorithm was successful in achieving an AUC of 0.7–0.9 in predicting the stage of cancer when using these radiomic attributes. Shao et al. [16] trained decision trees based on urinary metabolic markers to diagnose bladder cancer. They were able to achieve an accuracy of 76.6%, a sensitivity of 71.8%, and a precision of 86.6%. Ikeda et al. [17] used the technique of transfer learning, which enables anomaly detection by using gastroscopic images, to extract important features that apply to cystoscopic images. The dataset used contained 22 cystoscopic images, and the model was compared to results from actual urologists and medical students, who were divided into groups based on their expertise levels. The median time taken by the AI was 5 s as compared to 634 s by the group of observers and achieved 0.930 as the maximum score for Youden's index.

Table 2. Studies using AI to diagnose urothelial cancer.

Study	Application of the Study	Type of Study	Size of the Sample Used	Features Used for Training	Algorithms Used	Accuracy, %	Sensitivity, %	Specificity, %	AUC
Xu et al., 2017 [14]	Differentiate bladder tumor and bladder wall tissue by MRI	Retrospective	62 patients (62 cancerous regions and 62 bladder wall regions)	Radiomic MRI characteristics: 2D texture characteristics and 3D texture characteristics	SVM (2D)	70.16–78.23	-	-	0.72–0.83
					SVM (3D)	71.77–85.48	-	-	0.77–0.89
					RF (2D)	70.16–79.84	-	-	0.72–0.82
					RF (3D)	68.56–85.48	-	-	0.73–0.87
					SVM (RFE-selected optimal features)	87.9	90.3	85.5	0.90
Garapati et al., 2017 [15]	Forecast the stage of the disease based on CT urography	Retrospective	76 CT urography cases (84 bladder cancer lesions: 43 < T2; 41 ≥ T2)	Pathological stage, CT urography morphological features, and textural features	LDA (training set)	-	-	-	0.91
					LDA (testing set)				0.88
					SVM (training set)				0.91
					SVM (testing set)				0.89
					RF (training set)				0.89
					RF (testing set)				0.97
					NN (training set)				0.89
					NN (testing set)				0.92
Shao et al., 2017 [16]	Forecast whether the disease is present or not	Prospective	87 bladder cancer patients and 65 patients without bladder cancer	6 urine metabolite markers (spectral ions)	DT: testing	76.6	71.9	86.7	-
					DT: training (5-fold cross validation)	84.8	81.8	88.0	-
Ikeda et al., 2019 [17]	Detect tumors	Retrospective	422 cystoscopic images	Transfer learning using features extracted from gastroscopic images	CNN	-	96.5	96.5	-

Computed Tomography (CT); convolutional neural network (CNN).

3.4. Renal Cancer

Detection of renal cell cancer (RCC) in its early stages is crucial for its effective treatment, which can be clinically difficult once it spreads. Clinicians can use metabolomics data along with Raman spectra for building AI models, which are effective in the diagnosis of RCC during or before surgery (Table 3). Zheng et al. [18] attempted to identify RCC using a cluster of nuclear-magnetic-resonance-based serum metabolite biomarkers. The authors started with using ANNs to a group and categorized serum metabolites as healthy or RCC and then estimated the detection of RCC in patients individually. Furthermore,

ANNs were used for testing patients with RCC who had undergone nephrectomy. The expectation was that an individual patient who was previously classified as RCC would now be healthy after going through a nephrectomy. Haifler et al. [19] used shortwave Raman spectroscopy for distinguishing intra-operatively between healthy and malignant renal tissue. Training an AI model using Raman spectra from RCC and standard tissue samples could improve the identification of benign versus malignant tissue during surgery; the identification currently relies on a frozen section of the pathological specimen [19].

Table 3. Studies using AI to diagnose renal cancer.

Study	Application of the Study	Type of Study	Size of the Sample Used	Features Used for Training	Algorithms Used	Accuracy, %	Sensitivity, %	Specificity, %	AUC
Zheng et al., 2016 [18]	Forecast the presence of the disease in the earlier stages	Retrospective	126 patients (68 healthy participants and 48 renal cell cancer (RCC) patients)	Serum metabolome biomarker cluster	ANN: healthy participants	91.3	-	-	-
					ANN: RCC	94.7	-	-	-
Haifler et al., 2018 [19]	Discriminate between normal and malignant renal tissue	Prospective	6 clear-cell RCC specimens; 6 normal kidney tissue specimens	Short-wave infrared Raman spectroscopy	SMLR	92.5	95.8	88.8	0.94

Sparse Multinomial Logistic Regression (SMLR).

3.5. Hydronephrosis/Urinary Reflux

Radiomic imaging technologies are used along with AI to diagnose clinically relevant hydronephrosis and/or urinary reflex. Blum et al. [20] used ML techniques to create a model that is capable of detecting hydronephrosis based on renogram features. The analysis successfully displayed a higher precision in detecting hydronephrosis when compared with just half-time and 30 min clearance. Cerrolaza et al. [21] used ultrasound features to develop ML methods that help in predicting renal obstruction (halftime > 30 min). Logvinenko et al. [22] used ultrasonography results to estimate vesicoureteric reflux (VUR) on the emptying after the cystourethrogram. They found that the AI model worked marginally better than the multivariate logistic regression.

3.6. Reproductive Urology

Statistics reveal that around 70 million couples globally are failing to conceive, and male infertility is held responsible for 50% of these cases. Various factors contribute to reproductive problems in men, such as genetic mutations, lifestyle choices, and medical illnesses. Considering such factors, many investigators have paired predictive analytics with AI techniques in their studies to demonstrate how AI could be of assistance in reproductive urology. In the studies by Gil et al. [23] and Candemir et al. [24], AI networks and algorithmic models were used to predict semen quality by considering variables such as lifestyle and environmental factors. Both studies displayed high accuracies, the first study showing an accuracy of ~86% for sperm concentration and 73–76% for motility and the second showing an accuracy of ~90%. These predictive models for semen quality could certainly be used as a tool for screening men with fertility issues to effectively expose any underlying seminal disorders. Among the men, 10–20% undergoing infertility evaluation are found to be suffering from azoospermia, a medical condition in men that causes impotency due to inadequate or no sperm production [25]. Akinsal et al. performed a retrospective study to predict the subset of azoospermic patients that should undergo additional genetic evaluation by applying logistic regression analyses and ANNs [26]. The model identified azoospermic patients with chromosomal abnormalities and those without chromosomal abnormalities with an accuracy of 95%. Exploiting AI to identify individuals with potential genetic abnormalities may mitigate the expense and time lag of formal genetic testing. Apart from predicting semen quality, AI has also been applied in various investigations to determine potential biomarkers for infecundity. In a study by Vickram et al., three different models of ANNs were employed to predict the biochemical parameters for male infertility, of which the backpropagation neural network (BNN) showed minimum error [27]. Men with infertility issues are asked to undergo semen analysis in which most of the parameters, such as sperm motility and concentration, are measured manually. To avoid these time-consuming procedures and the available expensive alternate procedures,

Thirumalarjaju et al. introduced an AI-based approach using ANNs that was successful in producing the desired results in analyzing sperm morphology. The network identified abnormal semen samples with a staggering accuracy of 100% [28].

3.7. Urolithiasis

There has been a drastic alteration in the way urolithiasis cases are handled now compared with how they were handled in the past, and this approach will be highly influenced by AI techniques [29]. The future of AI in this field could provide complete management for urolithiasis: prevention, diagnosis, and treatment. Kazemi et al. [30] introduced a novel decision support system based on ensemble learning for the early detection (prevention) of kidney stones and explained the underlying mechanisms to determine the type of kidney stones. Various AI algorithms such as the Bayesian model, decision trees, ANNs, and rule-based classifiers were used in this system to understand the complex biological features involved in predicting kidney stones, with the system yielding an accuracy of 97.1%. Längkvist et al. [31] built a CNN (convolutional neural network) model for the detection of ureteral stones in high-resolution CT scans. This model was able to classify stones with a specificity of 100%, where the false positive was found to be 2.68 per scan and the AUC–ROC (receiver operating characteristic curve) was 0.9971.

3.8. Pediatric Urology

Pediatric urology handles congenital birth disabilities and disorders in newborn and young children. Though AI is yet to be wholly accepted and explored in this field, it certainly has brought new possibilities to light. About 1–3% of infants suffer from VUR, a condition that could potentially affect the bladder and kidneys if not diagnosed and treated earlier. One of the initial applications of AI in pediatric urology was the use of ANN architectures for the prognosis of VUR. To avoid a painful procedure for VUR detection, such as voiding cystourethrogram (VCUG), that exposes children to radiation, Papadopoulos et al. proposed an ML framework called Venn prediction for detecting VUR [32]. The model exhibited better sensitivity compared with other techniques. Likewise, another novel ML model was suggested to predict the future risk of febrile urinary tract infections (UTIs) related to VUR [33]. The predictive model performed with a reasonable degree of certainty in recognizing children most likely to benefit from VCUG, thus enabling personalized treatment.

3.9. Endourological Procedures

Endourology is another area in urology where AI is used to reach novel directions in planning and surgical interventions. Some of the previously mentioned minimally invasive procedures also come under this subfield. Images captured during cystoscopy play a pivotal role in the identification of bladder diseases. Ikeda et al. [17] introduced a support system based on CNNs for the proper diagnosis of bladder cancer using 2102 cystoscopic images. The built model separated the images of normal tissue from those of tumor lesions with high accuracy (area under ROC: 0.98; maximum Youden index (YI): 0.837; sensitivity: 89.7%; and specificity: 94%).

4. Outcomes Prediction

Patient outcome predictive analysis requires developing statistical methods that can interpret data to forecast outcomes for a particular patient. We can use either statistical modeling techniques or new methods emerging in the field of AI. These methods have the potential to handle the lack of accuracy and complexity that is typical in clinical and biological data. Additionally, AI techniques can handle the analysis of big data that are too big or too complex for standard statistical models more efficiently [34].

4.1. Prostate Cancer

Clinicopathological characteristics of individual patients are used to develop AI algorithms to forecast the outcome. Wong et al. [35] used clinicopathological characteristics of each patient to develop ML algorithms that can estimate the biochemical recurrence following prostatectomy (Table 4). They developed three different ML algorithms that were trained on a dataset of 338 patients to achieve an accuracy between 95% and 98% and an AUC between 0.9 and 0.94. In comparison to the conventional Cox regression analysis, these methods had better predictive efficiency. Tissue morphometric data [36], imaging radiomic features [37,38], and tissue genomic profiling [39,40] are also among the methods that are used for outcome forecasting of a patient. These studies have successfully demonstrated that AI has a higher accuracy when it comes to outcome prediction than other already existing methods.

Apart from the medical causes, surgical performance can also affect patient outcomes. Hung et al. [41,42] created and tested AI algorithms to find out the duration that a patient will have to stay in the hospital and the recovery of urinary control following robotic radical prostatectomy (Table 4). The algorithms were able to achieve an accuracy of 87.2% in the estimation of hospital stay and a C-index of 0.6 for estimating urinary control.

Table 4. Studies using AI to predict outcomes of prostate cancer.

Study	Application of the Study	Type of Study	Size of the Sample Used	Features Used for Training	Algorithms Used	Accuracy, %	Sensitivity, %	Specificity, %	C-index	AUC
Lam et al., 2014 [43]	Forecast mortality for a period of 5 years after radical cystectomy	Retrospective	117 patients (83 training, 17 validation, and 117 testing)	Age, tumor stage, albumin level, surgical approach	ANN	77.8	-	-	-	0.829
Wang et al., 2015 [44]	Forecast mortality for a period of 5 years after radical cystectomy	Retrospective	117 patients	Gender, age, age range, albumin, surgical approach 1/2, preoperative albumin, tumor stage, follow-up period, type of diversion	NN	72.2	77.6	68.1	-	-
					ELM	76.7	73.5	81.5	-	-
					RELM	80.0	85.6	72.4	-	-
					RBF	76.7	79.0	75.3	-	-
					SVM	75.6	75.4	77.0	-	-
					NB	73.3	73.8	73.4	-	-
					k-NN	72.2	75.1	70.1	-	-
Sapre et al., 2016 [45]	Predict urothelial carcinoma recurrence	Prospective	Training set 81 patients (21 benign controls, 30 no recurrence, and 30 active cancer recurrence); testing set 50 patients	Urinary miRNAs (miR205, miR34a, miR21, miR221, miR16, miR200c)	SVM (recurrence)	-	88.0	48.0	-	-
					SVM (tumor presence): training	-	-	-	-	0.85
					SVM (tumor presence): testing	-	-	-	-	0.74
					SVM (T1)	-	-	-	-	0.92
					SVM (Ta)	-	-	-	-	0.72
					SVM (T2,3,4)	-	-	-	-	0.73
					SVM (high volume)	-	-	-	-	0.81
					SVM (low volume)	-	-	-	-	0.69
					SVM (low grade)	-	-	-	-	0.76
					SVM (high grade)	-	-	-	-	0.75
					SVM (initial tumor)	-	-	-	-	0.76
Bartsch et al., 2016 [46]	Estimate the risk of recurrence in 5 years for non-muscle-invasive urothelial carcinoma after transurethral resection of the bladder	Retrospective	112 frozen non-muscle-invasive urothelial carcinoma specimens	Genes in DNA sampling	GP (3-gene rule): training	-	80.4	90.0	-	-
					GP (3-gene rule): testing	-	70.6	66.7	-	-
					GP (5-gene combined rule): training	-	77.1	84.6	-	-
					GP (5-gene combined rule): testing	-	68.6	61.5	-	-

Regularized Extreme Learning Machine (RELM); MicroRNA (miRNA); Glycoprotein (GP).

4.2. Urothelial Cancer

Urothelial cancers have a high chance of recurrence. AI systems for forecasting cancer recurrence and patient survival have been engineered [43–46] (Table 5). Lam et al. [43] and Wang et al. [44] used clinicopathological evidence to create and test a significant number of AI algorithms to estimate the 5-year survival after radical cystectomy. Their work results obtained are equivalent to those obtained by other statistical methods. Sapre et al. [45] proposed using an ML classifier with urinary microRNA to diagnose bladder cancer in patients. The classification results by this research achieved an AUC between 0.8 and 0.9 in observing a clinically relevant disease, while also reducing the requirement for cystoscopy by 30%. Bartsch et al. [46] used gene expression profiling to develop AI strategies to forecast the recurrence of non-muscle-invasive bladder cancer. Such experiments have demonstrated the possibility of the potential uses of AI for the treatment of urothelial carcinoma.

Table 5. Studies using AI to predict outcomes of urothelial cancer.

Study	Application of the Study	Type of Study	Size of the Sample Used	Features Used for Training	Algorithms Used	Accuracy, %	Sensitivity, %	Specificity, %	C-index	AUC
Wong et al., 2019 [ ]	Estimate the recurrence of the disease after radical prostatectomy	Prospective	338 patients	Patient clinicopathology information	k-NN	97.6	78.0	69.0	-	0.903
					RF	95.3	76.0	64.0	-	0.924
					LR	97.6	75.0	69.0	-	0.94
Harder et al., 2018 [ ]	Estimate the recurrence of the disease after radical prostatectomy	Retrospective	90 patients (40 with PSA recurrence)	Tissue phenomics of the disease	Hierarchical clustering	86.6	82.5	90.0	-	-
					naive Bayes	83.3	80.0	86.0	-	-
					classification and regression tree	83.3	70.0	94.0	-	-
					k-NN	85.5	80.0	90.0	-	-
					Linear predictor	87.8	94.0	80.0	-	-
					SVM (linear kernel)	86.7	77.5	94.0	-	-
					SVM (radial bias function kernel)	82.0	75	88.0	-	-
Zhang et al., 2016 [ ]	Estimate the recurrence of the disease after radical prostatectomy	Retrospective	205 patients (61 with biochemical recurrence)	Radiomic MRI characteristics	SVM	92.2	93.3	91.7	-	0.96
Shiradker et al., 2018 [ ]	Predict the biochemical recurrence of prostate cancer using MRI	Retrospective	120 patients (70 training; 50 validation)	Patient clinicopathological data and radiomic MRI characteristics	LDA (radiomic alone, training)	-	-	-	-	0.54
					SVM (radiomic alone, training)	-	-	-	-	0.84
					RF (radiomic alone, training)	-	-	-	-	0.52
					SVM (radiomic alone testing)	-	-	-	-	0.73
					SVM (radiomic + clinical training)	-	-	-	-	0.91
					SVM (radiomic + clinical testing)	-	-	-	-	0.74
Zhang et al. 2017 [ ]	Estimate biological recurrence after radical prostatectomy	Retrospective	424 patients (58 with recurrence)	Somatic gene mutation profiles	SVM (genetic signature alone)	66.2	-	-	-	0.7
					SVM (genetic signature + clinicopathological features)	71.3	-	-	-	0.75
Lalonde et al. 2014 [ ]	Predict the biochemical recurrence after radiation or radical prostatectomy	Retrospective	397 patients (126 training, 154 validation, and 117 testing)	Genes of the disease, general genomic instability, and tumor microenvironment	RF (validation set 1)	-	-	-	0.7	0.74
					RF (validation set 1)	-	-	-	0.74	0.84
					RF (validation set 2)	-	-	-	0.67	0.64
					RF (validation set 2)	-	-	-	0.73	0.75
Hung et al. 2018 [ ]	Predict the length of stay required in the hospital after radical prostatectomy	Ambispective	78 patients	25 surgical robotic APMs	RF	87.2	-	-	-	-
					RF (APMs and patient demographics)	88.5	-	-	-	-
					SVM	83.3	-	-	-	-
					LR	82.1	-	-	-	-
Hung et al. 2018 [ ]	Predict urinary continence recovery after robotic radical prostatectomy	Ambispective	79 patients	16 clinicopathological features and 492 robotic APMs	Random survival forests, Deep-learning-model-based survival analysis	-	-	-	0.58	-
						-	-	-	0.6	-

Automated Performance Metrics (APM).

4.3. Urolithiasis

Percutaneous nephrolithotomy (PCNL) and shockwave lithotripsy (SWL) are commonly recognized therapeutic methods for urolithiasis; however, the rates of success may differ significantly and might include repeat procedures in case the treatment is unsuccessful. Aminsharifi et al. [47] used ANNs to forecast a stone-free PCNL rate with an accuracy of 82.8% and the need to repeat PCNL with an accuracy of 97.7%. Mannil et al. [48] focused their study on the individual patient, using the patient's body mass index (BMI), along with the 3D texture and scale of the stone, also accounting for the skin-to-stone distance to estimate the performance of SWL. The authors developed and tested five AI algorithms, each with varying 3D textural permutations of patient characteristics, to register AUC values between 0.79 and 0.85, which was an increment from the AUC score of 0.58 that was achieved when using only patient characteristics. For a different report, 3D texture analysis was used to estimate the number of shock waves needed for effective SWL [49]. Against other statistical models, AI displays the most accurate predictions of the number of shock waves needed (<72 or ≥ 72), with an AUC of 0.838 recorded. Both of Mannil et al.'s [48,49] experiments demonstrated that using AI along with advanced textural analysis methods is practical, reproducible, and predictive of SWL performance.

4.4. Renal Transplant

With renal transplantation (RT) being the best available therapy for end-stage renal failure (ESRF), some hindrances are faced in the procedure that can be dealt with by analyzing the survival of transplant patients. The availability of medical data and improving AI techniques have made this challenging prospect more achievable.

The current trend of AI in RT revolves around ensemble learning, where multiple models are combined to achieve better predictive performance. Ethan et al. [50] proposed an ensemble model of ML algorithms for the effective allocation of kidneys by using 18 different predictive variables. The survival model exhibited a higher index of concordance (0.724) than the other existing models (0.68) used for determining recipient priority in the allocation system. Recently, a risk prediction score named iBox has been developed by an international team of French researchers for forecasting the risk of allograft failure after RT [51]. This robust system outperforms the current golden standard (estimated glomerular filtration rate and proteinuria) to monitor kidney recipients. The forecasts of this method, validated on more than 7500 patients, are extremely accurate in decision making, independent of the healthcare environment, medical conditions, clinical action, or actual patient treatment.

Though RT is a better option over dialysis, the recipient's kidney is always at a risk of rejection, and hence early identification of such complications is necessary. Abdeltawab et al. [52] came up with a non-invasive method for the timely diagnosis of acute RT rejection. The authors developed a novel deep-learning-based computer-aided diagnostic system drawn upon both imaging and clinical biomarkers. With its sensitivity of 93.3% and 92.3% specificity in distinguishing between non-rejected and discharged renal transplants, the proposed method produced an accuracy of 92.9%. Using RT survivor statistics, Kyung et al. [53] conducted a retrospective study and built a predictive model to evaluate graft survival in RT receivers. Their survival decision tree model performed better compared to the conventional decision tree and Cox regression models, with indexes of concordance of 0.80, 0.71, and 0.60–0.63, respectively.

5. Treatment Planning

5.1. Prostate Cancer Radiotherapy

Brachytherapy for prostate cancer involves a systematic preparation by a brachytherapist, a time-consuming process that can have varied results, depending on the observer [54]. There has been a high degree of research involving the use of ML algorithms to rapidly build recovery schedules for brachytherapy [54,55]. The time required to create and test the algorithms was found to be much shorter (0.8 vs. 17.9 min; $p = 0.002$), while the dosimetry metrics predicted were close to that of the qualified brachytherapist [55]. The accuracy of the dosimetry may be influenced because of different geometrical complexities during external radiotherapy. AI algorithms were developed by Guidi et al. [56] to handle such issues related to avoiding radiation injuries. CT images are used to train the AI algorithms in the radiotherapy planning and recovery phase of the treatment, which are used to compare scheduled and performed radiation therapy, helping patients who thereby benefit from receiving individualized care.

5.2. Cancer Drug Selection

AI interventions will be of assistance in the choice of adequate medications for cancer diagnosis and treatment. Saeed et al. [57] used ML technologies to measure and assess their activity with more than 300 forms of drugs in castration-resistant prostate cancer cells. Navitoclax family inhibitor Bcl-2 was described as highly active in patients with prostate cancer resistant to castration.

5.3. Surgical Skill Assessment

The evaluation of medical expertise and success is usually carried out by manual peer examination, allowing professionals to evaluate the surgical success or to monitor surgical performance. Such evaluations are often unreliable and increase the uncertainty due to different definitions of success by various observers. Endoscopic instruments offer direct visualization that is integrated with video cameras. These data, along with other types of information, including the movement of the surgical instruments, can also be collected. Such imagery and output data from the surgical robot can be used to test surgical output automatically using AI techniques. Figure 4 shows the procedural representation of a general biopsy using AI techniques. Anatomical landmark identification is an important metric in the assessment of advanced surgical skills. Nosrati et al. [58] and Baghdadi et al. [59] used ML algorithms to study the color and textural features from visualization of the surgical sites' anatomical features during partial nephrectomy and radical prostatectomy.

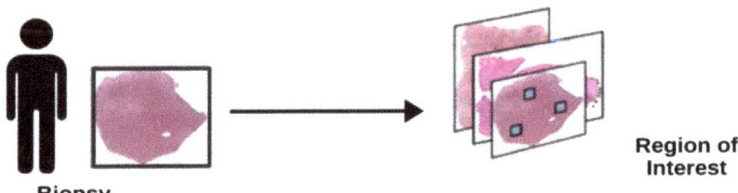

(a) Identification/Segmentation of region of interest

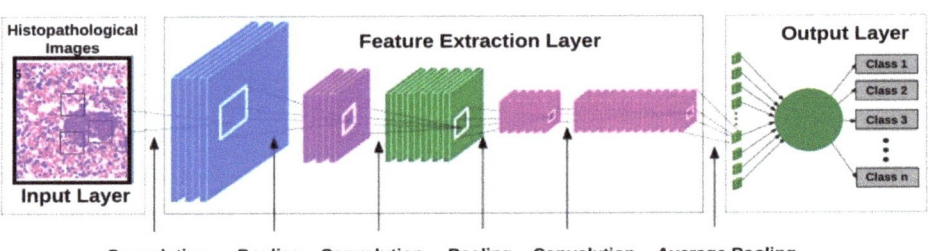

(b) Classification of histopathology images

Figure 4. (a) Identification/Segmentation of the region of interest. (b) Classification of histopathological images using a deep learning technique.

Tracking the movements and actions of the surgical instruments is also an important metric for performance assessment. Ghani et al. [60] looked at the movements of instruments to determine surgical skills and techniques. The authors collected data on the movements of the instruments either manually or by using motion trackers, which were then fed to an ML algorithm to determine the expertise level of the surgeon, achieving a precision between 83.3% and 100% [60].

6. Robotic Surgery

Apart from assessing the surgical skill, as discussed in the previous section, AI also plays a key role in improving new surgical techniques such as minimally invasive procedures involving surgical robots. Determining the best practices by analyzing the patterns and aiding in reducing technical errors are the primary tasks of AI in robotic surgery. Its performance in each sub-specialty of urology is discussed below.

6.1. Urologic Oncology

Recent advances in robotic urologic surgery and minimally invasive procedures have enabled approaches to treating prostate cancer, such as laparoscopic prostatectomy and robotic-assisted surgery. Robotic prostate surgery is an extremely precise procedure that provides excellent cancer control and is considered safe in experienced hands.

Radical cystectomy has been the surgical standard to treat patients suffering from muscle-invasive bladder cancer. Though there is a significant reduction in the estimated blood loss (EBL), the blood transfusion rate, and the length of stay in robotic-assisted radical cystectomy (RARC) compared to those in open radical cystectomy (ORC), the complications and the positive margin status have been found to be similar [61–68]. Although the role of RARC is controversial, it has become an acceptable alternative to open surgery by some guideline organizations, including the European Association of Urology [62].

6.2. Reproductive Urology

Etafy et al. [69], in a study, validated that robot-assisted microsurgical procedures are now safe and practicable in dealing with male infertility. More than 500,000 American men opt for vasectomy as a method of contraception annually, of which 2–6% will eventually undergo vasectomy reversal [70]. Studies have shown that robot-assisted vasovasostomy (RAVV) yields comparable results to that of the pure microsurgical technique [71]. Though the former approach is not superior, it offers a few additional advantages over normal surgical procedures. These benefits include the elimination of tremors, multiview magnification, additional instrument arms, and enhanced dexterity with articulating instrument arms.

6.3. Pediatric Urology

In pediatrics, robotic surgery remains controversial due to both cost and the lack of published high-level evidence. Ballouhey et al. [72] discussed how size difference in children cannot be a limiting factor for performing robotic surgery (patients with body weight of >15 kg or <15 kg yielded similar results). Robot-assisted laparoscopic pyeloplasty (RALP) is the standard treatment of ureteropelvic junction obstruction in older children and has even been performed in infants and redo procedures. In a study by Avery et al. [73], among the 60-patient cohort with a mean age of 7.3 months, 91% showed improvement or resolution of hydronephrosis after pyeloplasty, with 11% facing post-operative complications and 2 patients requiring redo procedures. Redo robotic pyeloplasty is deemed a safe and effective approach for recurring ureteropelvic junction obstruction, reporting up to 100% success rates and 0% complication rates [74]. Along with RALP (Robot-assisted laparoscopic pyeloplasty), robot assistance in nephrectomy [75], ureteroureterostomy [76], ureteral reimplantation [77], and other procedures has yielded affirmative results and unlocked new possibilities in the field of pediatric urology.

6.4. Renal Transplant

Robot-assisted RT (RART) is another application of AI that is highly recommended for obese and high-risk ESRF patients as it delivers low complication rates and excellent graft function over conventional surgery [78]. RART is considered to be a safe, feasible, and reproducible option when performed by surgeons with practice in both robotic and conventional RT surgery.

7. Discussion

In this article, we explored how AI can help us in the diagnosis, outcome prediction, and other treatment processes of urological diseases, even when provided with a heterogeneous and complex dataset. The growth in the granularity of data due to the huge spike in data collection over the recent years makes interpretation and pattern identification difficult for traditional statistical models, which are restricted by the limitation of using fixed correlations that work on the assumption that the data will have linear relationships. AI is much more robust and flexible when it comes to working with different data types and dealing with noise, missing data, and infrequent visits by the patient. It can even handle high-dimensionality data, while making minimum assumptions.

Although using AI can be tricky, the results and accuracy achieved when it is used correctly exceed those observed with the standard statistical models. It can also help in simplifying manually performed procedures and thus reducing the variation in outcomes due to human ability, bias, and methodological mistakes or inefficiencies. Therefore, AI-based models help clinicians in getting early, reliable, and personalized data that can help in the decision making.

It is observed that AI achieves a higher accuracy for most tasks, but it cannot be used to answer every question. Sometimes, standard statistical models can outperform AI models. Kattan et al. [79] compared ML estimation and Cox proportional risk regression methods based on three separate datasets of urological results. Cox regression could correspond with or surpass the ML model predictions. Neural networks have freely used parameters for the transformation of feature and class prediction, the neural networks being accurate and adapted to the maximal values of these free parameters. A well-constructed conventional model can outperform an ML model built lousily. Another issue with using ML-based models is something called a black box. When we make a deep neural network, the model builds non-linear, non-monotonic response functions, which despite having remarkable accuracy might be harder to explain, which makes the performance of these networks more empirical than theoretical.

Several clinicians and researchers have discussed the role of AI in healthcare and in treating certain urological conditions [80,81]. The approach adopted in this review provides a comprehensive view with an aim to address all possible aspects of AI in the field of urology. The studies reviewed by us vary in their training features, algorithms used, and the observed endpoints, which makes the task of quantitative analysis more difficult. In addition, these studies lack generalizability across different datasets as we have the results only for that particular dataset. Some of them also do not give a comparison with the standard statistical models, which limits our ability to understand how AI techniques are better than other models.

Real-life usage of AI technologies in the field of medicine is still a long way into the future. They face high levels of quality control and regulatory obstacles. The US FDA (United States Food and Drug Administration) has issued the first AI system assessment guidelines [82], which show that adaptive architecture should provide real-life evidence in clinical studies to assess the efficacy of AI techniques. AI models are data driven; they learn from the data that are given to them, and therefore require continuous training to maximize their utility and accuracy.

8. Conclusions

AI has come a long way in making exponential progress in healthcare over the past decade. There are still a lot of challenges and hurdles that need to be addressed before these techniques can be completely trusted to be used in the medical field. Though the future of AI in the field of urology is bright, considering it has already provided excellent solutions to handle various health issues through early diagnosis and personalized treatment, there is still a lot of room for improvement and growth when it comes to delivering solid results to positively influence more number of lives on an individualized basis.

Author Contributions: Concept and Study design: B.M.Z.H., B.K.S., N.N. and B.P.R.; Methods and experimental work: S.Z.R., H.K., R.P. and H.S.K.; Results analysis and conclusions: B.M.Z.H., B.K.S., N.N., R.P. and B.P.R.; Manuscript preparation: S.D.A.V.L., S.I., M.J.S. and D.K.S. All authors have read and agreed to the published version of the manuscript.

Funding: This research received no specific grant from any funding agency in the public, commercial, or not-for-profit sectors.

Institutional Review Board Statement: Not applicable.

Informed Consent Statement: Not applicable.

Data Availability Statement: Not applicable.

Conflicts of Interest: The authors declare that they have no conflict of interest.

References

1. Beam, A.L.; Kohane, I.S. Big Data and Machine Learning in Health Care. *JAMA* **2018**, *319*, 1317–1318. [CrossRef]
2. Kanagasingam, Y.; Xiao, D.; Vignarajan, J.; Preetham, A.; Tay-Kearney, M.-L.; Mehrotra, A. Evaluation of Artificial Intelligence–Based Grading of Diabetic Retinopathy in Primary Care. *JAMA Netw. Open* **2018**, *1*, e182665. [CrossRef]
3. Diprose, W.; Buist, N. Artificial intelligence in medicine: Humans need not apply? *New Zealand Med. J.* **2016**, *129*, 73–76. [PubMed]
4. Venkatramani, V. Urovision 2020: The future of urology. *Indian J. Urol.* **2015**, *31*, 150–155. [CrossRef] [PubMed]
5. Porpiglia, F.; Checcucci, E.; Amparore, D.; Piramide, F.; Volpi, G.; Granato, S.; Verri, P.; Manfredi, M.; Bellin, A.; Piazzolla, P.; et al. Three-dimensional Augmented Reality Robot-assisted Partial Nephrectomy in Case of Complex Tumours (PADUA $\geq$ 10): A New Intraoperative Tool Overcoming the Ultrasound Guidance. *Eur. Urol.* **2020**, *78*, 229–238. [CrossRef] [PubMed]
6. Kim, J.K.; Yook, I.H.; Choi, M.J.; Lee, J.S.; Park, Y.H.; Lee, J.Y.; Choi, I.Y. A Performance Comparison on the Machine Learning Classifiers in Predictive Pathology Staging of Prostate Cancer. *Stud. Health Technol. Inform.* **2017**, *245*, 1273.
7. Ms, A.A.; Viswanath, S.; Shiradkar, R.; Ghose, S.; Pahwa, S.; Moses, D.; Jambor, I.; Shnier, R.; Böhm, M.; Haynes, A.-M.; et al. Radiomic features on MRI enable risk categorization of prostate cancer patients on active surveillance: Preliminary findings. *J. Magn. Reson. Imaging* **2018**, *48*, 818–828. [CrossRef]
8. Ginsburg, S.B.; Ms, A.A.; Pahwa, S.; Gulani, V.; Ponsky, L.; Aronen, H.J.; Boström, P.J.; Böhm, M.; Haynes, A.-M.; Brenner, P.; et al. Radiomic features for prostate cancer detection on MRI differ between the transition and peripheral zones: Preliminary findings from a multi-institutional study. *J. Magn. Reson. Imaging* **2017**, *46*, 184–193. [CrossRef] [PubMed]
9. Merisaari, H.; Movahedi, P.; Perez, I.M.; Toivonen, J.; Pesola, M.; Taimen, P.; Boström, P.J.; Pahikkala, T.; Kiviniemi, A.; Aronen, H.J.; et al. Fitting methods for intravoxel incoherent motion imaging of prostate cancer on region of interest level: Repeatability and gleason score prediction. *Magn. Reson. Med.* **2016**, *77*, 1249–1264. [CrossRef]
10. Fehr, D.; Veeraraghavan, H.; Wibmer, A.; Gondo, T.; Matsumoto, K.; Vargas, H.A.; Sala, E.; Hricak, H.; Deasy, J.O. Automatic classification of prostate cancer Gleason scores from multiparametric magnetic resonance images. *Proc. Natl. Acad. Sci. USA* **2015**, *112*, E6265–E6273. [CrossRef]
11. Kwak, J.T.; Hewitt, S.M. Multiview boosting digital pathology analysis of prostate cancer. *Comput. Methods Programs Biomed.* **2017**, *142*, 91–99. [CrossRef] [PubMed]
12. Kwak, J.T.; Hewitt, S.M. Nuclear Architecture Analysis of Prostate Cancer via Convolutional Neural Networks. *IEEE Access* **2017**, *5*, 18526–18533. [CrossRef]
13. Nguyen, T.H.; Sridharan, S.; Macias, V.; Kajdacsy-Balla, A.; Melamed, J.; Do, M.N.; Popescu, G. Automatic Gleason grading of prostate cancer using quantitative phase imaging and machine learning. *J. Biomed. Opt.* **2017**, *22*, 036015. [CrossRef]
14. Xu, X.; Zhang, X.; Tian, Q.; Zhang, G.; Liu, Y.; Cui, G.; Meng, J.; Wu, Y.; Liu, T.; Yang, Z.; et al. Three-dimensional texture features from intensity and high-order derivative maps for the discrimination between bladder tumors and wall tissues via MRI. *Int. J. Comput. Assist. Radiol. Surg.* **2017**, *12*, 645–656. [CrossRef] [PubMed]
15. Garapati, S.S.; Hadjiiski, L.; Cha, K.H.; Chan, H.-P.; Caoili, E.M.; Cohan, R.H.; Weizer, A.; Alva, A.; Paramagul, C.; Wei, J.; et al. Urinary bladder cancer staging in CT urography using machine learning. *Med. Phys.* **2017**, *44*, 5814–5823. [CrossRef] [PubMed]

16. Shao, C.-H.; Chen, C.-L.; Lin, J.-Y.; Chen, C.-J.; Fu, S.-H.; Chen, Y.-T.; Chang, Y.-S.; Yu, J.-S.; Tsui, K.-H.; Juo, C.-G.; et al. Metabolite marker discovery for the detection of bladder cancer by comparative metabolomics. *Oncotarget* **2017**, *8*, 38802–38810. [CrossRef] [PubMed]
17. Ikeda, A.; Nosato, H.; Kochi, Y.; Kojima, T.; Kawai, K.; Sakanashi, H.; Murakawa, M.; Nishiyama, H. Support System of Cystoscopic Diagnosis for Bladder Cancer Based on Artificial Intelligence. *J. Endourol.* **2020**, *34*, 352–358. [CrossRef] [PubMed]
18. Zheng, H.; Ji, J.; Zhao, L.; Chen, M.; Shi, A.; Pan, L.; Huang, Y.; Zhang, H.; Dong, B.; Gao, H. Prediction and diagnosis of renal cell carcinoma using nuclear magnetic resonance-based serum metabolomics and self-organizing maps. *Oncotarget* **2016**, *7*, 59189–59198. [CrossRef]
19. Haifler, M.; Pence, I.; Sun, Y.; Kutikov, A.; Uzzo, R.G.; Mahadevan-Jansen, A.; Patil, C.A. Discrimination of malignant and normal kidney tissue with short wave infrared dispersive Raman spectroscopy. *J. Biophotonics* **2018**, *11*, e201700188. [CrossRef]
20. Blum, E.S.; Porras, A.R.; Biggs, E.; Tabrizi, P.R.; Sussman, R.D.; Sprague, B.M.; Shalaby-Rana, E.; Majd, M.; Pohl, H.G.; Linguraru, M.G. Early Detection of Ureteropelvic Junction Obstruction Using Signal Analysis and Machine Learning: A Dynamic Solution to a Dynamic Problem. *J. Urol.* **2018**, *199*, 847–852. [CrossRef]
21. Cerrolaza, J.J.; Peters, C.A.; Martin, A.D.; Myers, E.; Safdar, N.; Linguraru, M.G. Quantitative Ultrasound for Measuring Obstructive Severity in Children with Hydronephrosis. *J. Urol.* **2016**, *195*, 1093–1099. [CrossRef]
22. Logvinenko, T.; Chow, J.S.; Nelson, C.P. Predictive value of specific ultrasound findings when used as a screening test for abnormalities on VCUG. *J. Pediatr. Urol.* **2015**, *11*, 176.e1–176.e7. [CrossRef]
23. Gil, D.; Girela, J.L.; De Juan, J.; Gomez-Torres, M.J.; Johnsson, M. Predicting seminal quality with artificial intelligence methods. *Expert Syst. Appl.* **2012**, *39*, 12564–12573. [CrossRef]
24. Candemir, C. Estimating the Semen Quality from Life-Style Using Fuzzy Radial Basis Functions. *Int. J. Mach. Learn. Comput.* **2018**, *8*, 44–48. [CrossRef]
25. Luchey, A.M.; Agarwal, G.; Poch, M.A. Robotic-Assisted Radical Cystectomy. *Cancer Control.* **2015**, *22*, 301–306. [CrossRef] [PubMed]
26. Akinsal, E.C.; Haznedar, B.; Baydilli, N.; Kalinli, A.; Ozturk, A.; Ekmekçioğlu, O. Artificial Neural Network for the Prediction of Chromosomal Abnormalities in Azoospermic Males. *Urol. J.* **2018**, *15*, 122–125.
27. Vickram, A.S.; Kamini, A.R.; Das, R.; Pathy, M.R.; Parameswari, R.; Archana, K.; Sridharan, T.B. Validation of artificial neural network models for predicting biochemical markers associated with male infertility. *Syst. Biol. Reprod. Med.* **2016**, *62*, 258–265. [CrossRef] [PubMed]
28. Thirumalaraju, P.; Bormann, C.; Kanakasabapathy, M.; Doshi, F.; Souter, I.; Dimitriadis, I.; Shafiee, H. Automated sperm morpshology testing using artificial intelligence. *Fertil. Steril.* **2018**, *110*, e432. [CrossRef]
29. Shah, M.; Naik, N.; Somani, B.K.; Hameed, B.M.Z. Artificial intelligence (AI) in urology-Current use and future directions: An iTRUE study. *Türk Urol. Derg. Turk. J. Urol.* **2020**, *46*, S27–S39. [CrossRef]
30. Kazemi, Y.; Mirroshandel, S.A. A novel method for predicting kidney stone type using ensemble learning. *Artif. Intell. Med.* **2018**, *84*, 117–126. [CrossRef]
31. Längkvist, M.; Jendeberg, J.; Thunberg, P.; Loutfi, A.; Lidén, M. Computer aided detection of ureteral stones in thin slice computed tomography volumes using Convolutional Neural Networks. *Comput. Biol. Med.* **2018**, *97*, 153–160. [CrossRef]
32. Papadopoulos, H.; Anastassopoulos, G. Probabilistic Prediction for the Detection of Vesicoureteral Reflux. *Program. Ing. Nat.* **2013**, *383*, 253–262. [CrossRef]
33. Advanced Analytics Group of Pediatric Urology and ORC Personalized Medicine Group. Targeted Workup after Initial Febrile Urinary Tract Infection: Using a Novel Machine Learning Model to Identify Children Most Likely to Benefit from Voiding Cystourethrogram. *J. Urol.* **2019**, *202*, 144–152. [CrossRef]
34. Cosma, G.; Brown, D.; Archer, M.; Khan, M.; Pockley, A.G. A survey on computational intelligence approaches for predictive modeling in prostate cancer. *Expert Syst. Appl.* **2017**, *70*, 1–19. [CrossRef]
35. Wong, N.C.; Lam, C.; Patterson, L.; Shayegan, B. Use of machine learning to predict early biochemical recurrence after robot-assisted prostatectomy. *BJU Int.* **2019**, *123*, 51–57. [CrossRef] [PubMed]
36. Harder, N.; Athelogou, M.; Hessel, H.; Brieu, N.; Yigitsoy, M.; Zimmermann, J.; Baatz, M.; Buchner, A.; Stief, C.G.; Kirchner, T.; et al. Tissue Phenomics for prognostic biomarker discovery in low- and intermediate-risk prostate cancer. *Sci. Rep.* **2018**, *8*, 1–19. [CrossRef]
37. Zhang, Y.-D.; Wang, J.; Wu, C.-J.; Bao, M.-L.; Li, H.; Wang, X.-N.; Tao, J.; Shi, H.-B. An imaging-based approach predicts clinical outcomes in prostate cancer through a novel support vector machine classification. *Oncotarget* **2016**, *7*, 78140–78151. [CrossRef]
38. Shiradkar, R.; Ghose, S.; Jambor, I.; Taimen, P.; Ettala, O.; Purysko, A.S.; Madabhushi, A. Radiomic features from pretreatment biparametric MRI predict prostate cancer biochemical recurrence: Preliminary findings. *J. Magn. Reson. Imaging* **2018**, *48*, 1626–1636. [CrossRef]
39. Zhang, S.; Xu, Y.; Hui, X.; Yang, F.; Hu, Y.; Shao, J.; Liang, H.; Wang, Y. Improvement in prediction of prostate cancer prognosis with somatic mutational signatures. *J. Cancer* **2017**, *8*, 3261–3267. [CrossRef]
40. Lalonde, E.; Ishkanian, A.S.; Sykes, J.; Fraser, M.; Ross-Adams, H.; Erho, N.; Dunning, M.J.; Halim, S.; Lamb, A.D.; Moon, N.C.; et al. Tumour genomic and microenvironmental heterogeneity for integrated prediction of 5-year biochemical recurrence of prostate cancer: A retrospective cohort study. *Lancet Oncol.* **2014**, *15*, 1521–1532. [CrossRef]

41. Atug, F.; Sanli, O.; Duru, A.D. Editorial Comment on: Utilizing Machine Learning and Automated Performance Metrics to Evaluate Robot-Assisted Radical Prostatectomy Performance and Predict Outcomes by Hung et al. *J. Endourol.* **2018**, *32*, 445. [CrossRef] [PubMed]
42. Hung, A.J.; Chen, J.; Ghodoussipour, S.; Oh, P.J.; Liu, Z.; Nguyen, J.; Purushotham, S.; Gill, I.S.; Liu, Y. A deep-learning model using automated performance metrics and clinical features to predict urinary continence recovery after robot-assisted radical prostatectomy. *BJU Int.* **2019**, *124*, 487–495. [CrossRef] [PubMed]
43. Lam, K.-M.; He, X.-J.; Choi, K.-S. Using artificial neural network to predict mortality of radical cystectomy for bladder cancer. In Proceedings of the 2014 International Conference on Smart Computing, Hong Kong, China, 3–5 November 2014; pp. 201–207.
44. Wang, G.; Lam, K.-M.; Deng, Z.; Choi, K.-S. Prediction of mortality after radical cystectomy for bladder cancer by machine learning techniques. *Comput. Biol. Med.* **2015**, *63*, 124–132. [CrossRef] [PubMed]
45. Sapre, N.; MacIntyre, G.; Clarkson, M.; Naeem, H.; Cmero, M.; Kowalczyk, A.; Anderson, P.D.; Costello, A.J.; Corcoran, N.M.; Hovens, C.M. A urinary microRNA signature can predict the presence of bladder urothelial carcinoma in patients undergoing surveillance. *Br. J. Cancer* **2016**, *114*, 454–462. [CrossRef]
46. Bartsch, G.; Mitra, A.P.; Mitra, S.A.; Almal, A.A.; Steven, K.E.; Skinner, D.G.; Fry, D.W.; Lenehan, P.F.; Worzel, W.P.; Cote, R.J. Use of Artificial Intelligence and Machine Learning Algorithms with Gene Expression Profiling to Predict Recurrent Nonmuscle Invasive Urothelial Carcinoma of the Bladder. *J. Urol.* **2016**, *195*, 493–498. [CrossRef]
47. Aminsharifi, A.; Irani, D.; Pooyesh, S.; Parvin, H.; Dehghani, S.; Yousofi, K.; Fazel, E.; Zibaie, F. Artificial Neural Network System to Predict the Postoperative Outcome of Percutaneous Nephrolithotomy. *J. Endourol.* **2017**, *31*, 461–467. [CrossRef]
48. Mannil, M.; Von Spiczak, J.; Hermanns, T.; Poyet, C.; Alkadhi, H.; Fankhauser, C.D. Three-Dimensional Texture Analysis with Machine Learning Provides Incremental Predictive Information for Successful Shock Wave Lithotripsy in Patients with Kidney Stones. *J. Urol.* **2018**, *200*, 829–836. [CrossRef]
49. Mannil, M.; Von Spiczak, J.; Hermanns, T.; Alkadhi, H.; Fankhauser, C.D. Prediction of successful shock wave lithotripsy with CT: A phantom study using texture analysis. *Abdom. Radiol.* **2017**, *43*, 1432–1438. [CrossRef]
50. Karthik, L.; Kumar, G.; Keswani, T.; Bhattacharyya, A.; Chandar, S.S.; Rao, K.V.B. Protease Inhibitors from Marine Actinobacteria as a Potential Source for Antimalarial Compound. *PLoS ONE* **2014**, *9*, e90972. [CrossRef]
51. Loupy, A.; Aubert, O.; Orandi, B.J.; Naesens, M.; Bouatou, Y.; Raynaud, M.; Divard, G.; Jackson, A.M.; Viglietti, D.; Giral, M.; et al. Prediction system for risk of allograft loss in patients receiving kidney transplants: International derivation and validation study. *BMJ* **2019**, *366*, l4923. [CrossRef]
52. Abdeltawab, H.; Shehata, M.; Shalaby, A.; Khalifa, F.; Mahmoud, A.; El-Ghar, M.A.; Dwyer, A.C.; Ghazal, M.; Hajjdiab, H.; Keynton, R.; et al. A Novel CNN-Based CAD System for Early Assessment of Transplanted Kidney Dysfunction. *Sci. Rep.* **2019**, *9*, 1–11. [CrossRef]
53. Yoo, K.D.; Noh, J.; Lee, H.; Kim, D.K.; Lim, C.S.; Kim, Y.H.; Lee, J.P.; Kim, G.; Kim, Y.S. A Machine Learning Approach Using Survival Statistics to Predict Graft Survival in Kidney Transplant Recipients: A Multicenter Cohort Study. *Sci. Rep.* **2017**, *7*, 1–12. [CrossRef]
54. Nouranian, S.; Ramezani, M.; Spadinger, I.; Morris, W.J.; Salcudean, S.E.; Abolmaesumi, P. Learning-Based Multi-Label Segmentation of Transrectal Ultrasound Images for Prostate Brachytherapy. *IEEE Trans. Med. Imaging* **2015**, *35*, 921–932. [CrossRef]
55. Nicolae, A.; Morton, G.; Chung, H.; Loblaw, A.; Jain, S.; Mitchell, D.; Lu, L.; Helou, J.; Al-Hanaqta, M.; Heath, E.; et al. Evaluation of a Machine-Learning Algorithm for Treatment Planning in Prostate Low-Dose-Rate Brachytherapy. *Int. J. Radiat. Oncol.* **2017**, *97*, 822–829. [CrossRef]
56. Guidi, G.; Maffei, N.; Vecchi, C.; Gottardi, G.; Ciarmatori, A.; Mistretta, G.M.; Mazzeo, E.; Giacobazzi, P.; Lohr, F.; Costi, T. Expert system classifier for adaptive radiation therapy in prostate cancer. *Australas. Phys. Eng. Sci. Med.* **2017**, *40*, 337–348. [CrossRef]
57. Saeed, K.; Rahkama, V.; Eldfors, S.; Bychkov, D.; Mpindi, J.P.; Yadav, B.; Paavolainen, L.; Aittokallio, T.; Heckman, C.; Wennerberg, K.; et al. Comprehensive Drug Testing of Patient-derived Conditionally Reprogrammed Cells from Castration-resistant Prostate Cancer. *Eur. Urol.* **2017**, *71*, 319–327. [CrossRef]
58. Nosrati, M.S.; Amir-Khalili, A.; Peyrat, J.-M.; Abi-Nahed, J.; Al-Alao, O.; Al-Ansari, A.; Abugharbieh, R.; Hamarneh, G. Endoscopic scene labelling and augmentation using intraoperative pulsatile motion and colour appearance cues with preoperative anatomical priors. *Int. J. Comput. Assist. Radiol. Surg.* **2016**, *11*, 1409–1418. [CrossRef]
59. Baghdadi, A.; Cavuoto, L.; Hussein, A.A.; Ahmed, Y.; Guru, K. PD58-04 Modeling Automated Assessment of Surgical Performance Utilizing Computer Vision: Proof of Concept. *J. Urol.* **2018**, *199*, e1134–e1135. [CrossRef]
60. Ghani, K.; Liu, Y.; Law, H.; He, D.; Miller, D.; Montie, J.; Deng, J. Video analysis of skill and technique (VAST): Machine learning to assess the technical skill of surgeons performing robotic prostatectomy. *Eur. Urol. Suppl.* **2017**, *16*, e1927–e1928. [CrossRef]
61. Sathianathen, N.J.; Kalapara, A.; Frydenberg, M.; Lawrentschuk, N.; Weight, C.J.; Parekh, D.; Konety, B.R. Robotic Assisted Radical Cystectomy vs Open Radical Cystectomy: Systematic Review and Meta-Analysis. *J Urol.* **2019**, *201*, 715–720. [CrossRef]
62. Witjes, J.A.; Lebret, T.; Compérat, E.M.; Cowan, N.C.; De Santis, M.; Bruins, H.M.; Hernández, V.; Espinós, E.L.; Dunn, J.; Rouanne, M.; et al. Updated 2016 EAU Guidelines on Muscle-invasive and Metastatic Bladder Cancer. *Eur. Urol.* **2017**, *71*, 462–475. [CrossRef] [PubMed]
63. Koelzer, V.H.; Rothschild, S.I.; Zihler, D.; Wicki, A.; Willi, B.; Willi, N.; Voegeli, M.; Cathomas, G.; Zippelius, A.; Mertz, K.D. Systemic inflammation in a melanoma patient treated with immune checkpoint inhibitors—An autopsy study. *J. Immunother. Cancer* **2016**, *4*, 13. [CrossRef] [PubMed]

64. Rai, B.P.; Bondad, J.; Vasdev, N.; Adshead, J.; Lane, T.; Ahmed, K.; Khan, M.S.; Dasgupta, P.; Guru, K.; Chlosta, P.L.; et al. Robotic versus open radical cystectomy for bladder cancer in adults. *Cochrane Database Syst Rev.* **2019**, *4*, CD011903. [CrossRef]
65. *Machine Learning in Medical Imaging*; Springer: Berling, Germany, 2017.
66. Kocak, B.; Yardimci, A.H.; Bektas, C.T.; Turkcanoglu, M.H.; Erdim, C.; Yucetas, U.; Koca, S.B.; Kilickesmez, O. Textural differences between renal cell carcinoma subtypes: Machine learning-based quantitative computed tomography texture analysis with independent external validation. *Eur. J. Radiol.* **2018**, *107*, 149–157. [CrossRef]
67. Han, S.; Hwang, S.I.; Lee, H.J. The Classification of Renal Cancer in 3-Phase CT Images Using a Deep Learning Method. *J. Digit. Imaging* **2019**, *32*, 638–643. [CrossRef]
68. Mastroianni, R.; Tuderti, G.; Anceschi, U.; Bove, A.M.; Brassetti, A.; Ferriero, M.; Zampa, A.; Giannarelli, D.; Guaglianone, S.; Gallucci, M.; et al. Comparison of Patient-reported Health-related Quality of Life Between Open Radical Cystectomy and Robot-assisted Radical Cystectomy with Intracorporeal Urinary Diversion: Interim Analysis of a Randomised Controlled Trial. *Eur. Urol. Focus* **2021**, S2405–S4569, 00059-6. [CrossRef]
69. Etafy, M.; Gudeloglu, A.; Brahmbhatt, J.V.; Parekattil, S.J. Review of the role of robotic surgery in male infertility. *Arab. J. Urol.* **2018**, *16*, 148–156. [CrossRef]
70. Kirby, E.W.; Hockenberry, M.; Lipshultz, L.I. Vasectomy reversal: Decision making and technical innovations. *Transl. Androl. Urol.* **2017**, *6*, 753–760. [CrossRef]
71. Parekattil, S.J.; Gudeloglu, A. Robotic assisted andrological surgery. *Asian J. Androl.* **2013**, *15*, 67–74. [CrossRef]
72. Ballouhey, Q.; Villemagne, T.; Cros, J.; Szwarc, C.; Braik, K.; Longis, B.; Lardy, H.; Fourcade, L. A comparison of robotic surgery in children weighing above and below 15.0 kg: Size does not affect surgery success. *Surg. Endosc.* **2014**, *29*, 2643–2650. [CrossRef]
73. Avery, D.I.; Herbst, K.W.; Lendvay, T.S.; Noh, P.H.; Dangle, P.; Gundeti, M.S.; Steele, M.C.; Corbett, S.T.; Peters, C.A.; Kim, C. Robot-assisted laparoscopic pyeloplasty: Multi-institutional experience in infants. *J. Pediatr. Urol.* **2015**, *11*, 139.e1–139.e5. [CrossRef]
74. Asensio, M.; Gander, R.; Royo, G.F.; Lloret, J. Failed pyeloplasty in children: Is robot-assisted laparoscopic reoperative repair feasible? *J. Pediatr. Urol.* **2015**, *11*, 69.e1–69.e6. [CrossRef]
75. Lee, R.S.; Sethi, A.S.; Passerotti, C.C.; Retik, A.B.; Borer, J.G.; Nguyen, H.T.; Peters, C.A. Robot Assisted Laparoscopic Partial Nephrectomy: A Viable and Safe Option in Children. *J. Urol.* **2009**, *181*, 823–829. [CrossRef]
76. Bowen, D.K.; Casey, J.T.; Cheng, E.Y.; Gong, E.M. Robotic-assisted laparoscopic transplant-to-native ureteroureterostomy in a pediatric patient. *J. Pediatr. Urol.* **2014**, *10*, 1284.e1–1284.e2. [CrossRef]
77. Marchini, G.S.; Hong, Y.K.; Minnillo, B.J.; Diamond, D.A.; Houck, C.S.; Meier, P.M.; Passerotti, C.C.; Kaplan, J.R.; Retik, A.B.; Nguyen, H.T. Robotic Assisted Laparoscopic Ureteral Reimplantation in Children: Case Matched Comparative Study with Open Surgical Approach. *J. Urol.* **2011**, *185*, 1870–1875. [CrossRef]
78. Breda, A.; Territo, A.; Gausa, L.; Tuğcu, V.; Alcaraz, A.; Musquera, M.; Decaestecker, K.; Desender, L.; Stockle, M.; Janssen, M.; et al. Robot-assisted Kidney Transplantation: The European Experience. *Eur. Urol.* **2018**, *73*, 273–281. [CrossRef]
79. French, A.; Lendvay, T.S.; Sweet, R.M.; Kowalewski, T.M. Predicting surgical skill from the first N seconds of a task: Value over task time using the isogony principle. *Int. J. Comput. Assist. Radiol. Surg.* **2017**, *12*, 1161–1170. [CrossRef]
80. Checcucci, E.; De Cillis, S.; Granato, S.; Chang, P.; Afyouni, A.S.; Okhunov, Z. Applications of neural networks in urology. *Curr. Opin. Urol.* **2020**, *30*, 788–807. [CrossRef]
81. Checcucci, E.; Autorino, R.; Cacciamani, G.E.; Amparore, D.; De Cillis, S.; Piana, A.; Piazzolla, P.; Vezzetti, E.; Fiori, C.; Veneziano, D.; et al. Artificial intelligence and neural networks in urology: Current clinical applications. *Minerva Urol. Nefrol.* **2020**, *72*, 49–57. [CrossRef]
82. Commissioner of the U.S. Food and Drug Administration. FDA Releases Artificial Intelligence/Machine Learning Action Plan. Available online: https://www.fda.gov/news-events/press-announcements/fda-releases-artificial-intelligencemachine-learning-action-plan (accessed on 6 March 2021).

MDPI
St. Alban-Anlage 66
4052 Basel
Switzerland
Tel. +41 61 683 77 34
Fax +41 61 302 89 18
www.mdpi.com

Journal of Clinical Medicine Editorial Office
E-mail: jcm@mdpi.com
www.mdpi.com/journal/jcm